THE MALNOURISHED MIND

It is a rare scientist who can communicate to the layman his broad insight into pervasive issues involving science and society. Dr. Elie A. Shneour is such a scientist. He is an internationally known neurochemist with extensive research, teaching, writing, and administrative experience. Dr. Shneour is a graduate of Columbia University (Bard College) and holds advanced degrees from the University of California at Berkeley and the School of Medicine at UCLA. He coauthored the critically acclaimed *Life Beyond the Earth,* and edited a major anthology and bibliography on *Biology and the Exploration of Mars* for the National Academy of Sciences. Dr. Shneour was on the research staff at Stanford University Medical Center, served as Associate Professor of Biology at the University of Utah for four years, and spent two years at the City of Hope National Medical Center's Division of Neurosciences before joining Calbiochem as its Director of Research. Dr. Shneour is a member of many professional societies, including the American Society for Neurochemistry, the International Society for Neurochemistry, the American Society of Biological Chemists, the Society for Neuroscience, and the New York Academy of Sciences. He resides in La Jolla, California, with his wife and two teen-aged sons.

THE
Malnourished Mind

ELIE A. SHNEOUR

Foreword by LEE SALK

ANCHOR PRESS/DOUBLEDAY

GARDEN CITY, NEW YORK, 1974

ISBN: 0-385-03909-3

Library of Congress Catalog Card Number: 73-9175

Copyright © 1974 by Elie A. Shneour

Printed in the United States of America

First Edition

for MARK and ALAN

FOREWORD

Dr. Shneour is not an alarmist. However, he presents some very alarming facts and formulations that have implications for the future of our civilization.

Dr. Shneour ranks among those of us who are concerned now —not when it is too late. In presenting his major thesis, that early-life malnutrition is an important element in shaping man's cognitive potential, he recognizes that we may not have all the information we might like to have at this time. He believes, however, that if we wait until all the evidence is available in complete detail, it will be too late for action. Existing evidence is suggestive enough to warrant action *now*.

It seems ironic that one should have to mobilize all kinds of evidence to make the point that feeding human beings is a worthwhile effort. We should need no *new* evidence that hunger and malnutrition are evil. Sometimes when scientific break-throughs are made, it is necessary to provide evidence that there will be no negative side effects to a new or recommended treatment before it is acceptable. Dr. Shneour's thesis that malnutrition during critical developmental stages is hazardous needs no documentation of possible negative side effects. Clearly, there can be no negative side effects to adequate nutrition; yet those

of us concerned with these problems are up against a great deal
of resistance in gaining recognition of the importance of this
problem that Dr. Shneour puts forth so comprehensively in his
book.

His book is a unique presentation of information from a wide
range of scientific disciplines. He is courageous in the presentation of his point of view; he draws freely, yet selectively, from
a wide range of information. While some may find it difficult
to justify the transition he makes from one discipline to another,
it is undeniable that he forces us to think of the long-range implications of the problem of malnutrition on the potential of
human behavior. I believe it is necessary to take this kind of
forceful approach, because so many of us find it hard, if not impossible, to identify with the problem of hunger and malnutrition. Somehow we view it as a problem that applies to other
people—oftentimes, "undesirables." It is far easier for us to concern ourselves with other health problems, such as cancer and
heart disease, since these are more threatening to the more liter-
ate, middle class of our culture.

In his selection of scientific information and in the development of his ideas, Dr. Shneour has formulated his viewpoint
on the problems of malnutrition during pregnancy and malnutrition during early life. These are problems of great magnitude
that have been severely neglected in spite of compelling evidence that deficiencies during early development can never be
made up later on. Our neglect of this problem may be causing
irreversible damage to developing nervous systems and prevent-
ing human beings in a large segment of this world from ever
reaching their cognitive potential.

Dr. Shneour is an advocate of children. He believes, as do I,
that the future of our civilization depends upon our providing
the children of today with the optimal conditions for healthy
physical and psychological growth. He acknowledges the idea of
the critical-period concept, a concept that is oftentimes ignored
by people in the behavioral and biological sciences. He recog-

nizes that ignoring the critical nature of certain developmental stages regarding human development can be hazardous. Moreover, he believes that prevention is the only answer when dealing with certain problems, such as the one he devotes himself to in this book.

The behavior of human beings in generations to come can be substantially influenced by the massive problem of malnutrition affecting people throughout this world. Most of us would like to believe this problem is far from home. It is not.

In viewing the vast number of books published annually on nutrition and diet, it is surprising that so many people blindly follow recommendations made by self-styled experts on the subject, whose advice is based upon views that are totally unscientific. Anyone concerned with nutrition and dieting should read Dr. Shneour's scientifically sound book for a perspective on the subject that no other book concerned with nutrition has ever offered. He discusses a range of subjects and theories from enzymes to Piaget, from the wild boy of Aveyron to intelligence tests, from the discovery of vitamins to the intrauterine environment. He wanders through various fields of information, much to the benefit of those who have never been exposed to the basic concepts of those disciplines, leaving the reader with a well-distilled body of information in all these areas.

Governmental agencies have paid lip service to, and set up committees to investigate, the existence of malnutrition, but they have done very little to alleviate the problem. Many legislators address themselves to problems of immediate concern to their constituency and that can be solved during their tenure in office. Unfortunately, the problem of malnutrition does not fit that category.

Only through educating more and more people about malnutrition and its effects and consequences on a wide scale, can we hope to put pressure on our legislators to do something about this enormous problem. Dr. Shneour has taken a giant step in this direction, and, hopefully, this material will be read not only by the lay public, but as well by every legislator who has it within his or her potential to engage in some social or legislative action toward its elimination.

Dr. Lee Salk

Professor of Pediatrics and Psychology
Cornell University College of Medicine

Director of Pediatric Psychology
The New York Hospital—Cornell Medical Center

CONTENTS

PREFACE

It is easy to generate a controversy where none has existed before. Simply pit in a public forum an articulate person committed to a given point of view against one holding an opposing view. It does not matter whether either of the protagonists is genuinely knowledgeable in the subject at issue. An appearance of conflicting authority is sufficient to suggest a meaningful difference of opinion between experts.

This book was written to review pertinent information on early-life malnutrition and its consequences on human cognition, a subject that readily lends itself to controversy. I have written it for the general reader, not the specialist, because only an informed public can ultimately influence the course of human events. All substantive statements made in this book are supported by references to the scientific literature, so that the reader may examine the information at its source instead of accepting at face value what I have written. Thus he may join the current healthy trend toward increased skepticism of the pronouncements and judgments of the so-called expert. I wish that more politicians would agree with David Ben-Gurion's statement, "Experts are all experts in things that have already happened; there are no experts in things that have never happened."[1]

---

[1] C. Legum, "The Most Revered Jew in the World," reprinted from the London *Observer*, by the Los Angeles *Times*, May 13, 1973, part IV, p. 3.

This applies particularly well to scientific and technological matters. Scientific knowledge derives its power not from authority but from reason. It is open to all who are willing to observe carefully and to reason from premise to conclusion. Science is among the most equalitarian of all human endeavors.

The idea for this book was born in January 1965 at Stanford University during an extraordinary discussion that included Professor William B. Shockley of Stanford's Department of Engineering Science, Dr. Irving Bengelsdorf, then Science Editor of the Los Angeles *Times*, Samuel Moffat, then Information Officer of the Stanford Medical Center, and the author, then with the Department of Genetics at Stanford University School of Medicine. A few days earlier, on January 7, 1965, Dr. Shockley had delivered the Nobel lecture at Gustavus Adolfus College, in Minnesota, on genetics and the future of man. In his talk Dr. Shockley expressed concern about the possible genetic deterioration of mankind through the selective multiplication of the less-gifted members of society. He proposed the imposition of a limitation on food supply and other resources to provoke a healthy competition between men to allow the fittest among them to survive. A storm of controversy followed this lecture.

While I disagree with Dr. Shockley's simplistic position, I am grateful to him for having provided the original impetus for writing this book. *The Malnourished Mind* is not a rebuttal. It is rather an assessment of the evidence that bears on early-life malnutrition, a critical part of the overall issue which emphasizes how complex are the problems of human survival.

An immense amount of information is available on this subject. The greatest challenge in the preparation of the manuscript was to make a judicious and balanced selection from that information. It was then necessary to weave the data into a meaningful pattern, tell a coherent story, and express a judgment on its probable significance. In the process, I have avoided complex technical arguments (concerning, for example, the g factor, heritability, minimum nutritional requirements), because they do not of themselves contribute useful insight into the problems encompassed by this book.

In describing specific examples of experimental work, I have retained the investigators' own words wherever possible, in order to avoid changes in the meaning conveyed in the original reports.

Many persons have contributed to the preparation of the manuscript. My wife Joan and I have worked as a close team throughout the endeavor. Her unrelenting analysis of the text is to a large degree responsible for any lucidity of expression I have achieved. She also did much of the library research, editing, and the ever-required typing. For the title I am indebted to my thirteen-year-old son Mark.

I owe a particularly heavy debt of gratitude to the following of my distinguished colleagues who reviewed specific chapters of this book and offered invaluable advice and criticism:

Samuel Barondes, Professor of Psychiatry, School of Medicine, University of California at San Diego; Walter F. Bodmer, Professor of Genetics, Genetics Laboratory, Department of Biochemistry, Oxford University, Oxford, England; Joaquín Cravioto, Scientific Research Division, Hospital del Niño, Institución Mexicana de Asistencia a la Niñez, México, D.F.; Gerard M. Lehrer, Professor of Neurology, Mount Sinai School of Medicine, City University of New York, New York, New York; I. Michael Lerner, Professor of Genetics, Department of Genetics, University of California at Berkeley, California; James L. McGaugh, Professor and Chairman of the Department of Psychobiology, University of California at Irvine, California; Richard and Cynthia Wimer, Division of Neurosciences, City of Hope National Medical Center, Duarte, California; Myron Winick, Professor of Nutrition and Director, Institute of Human Nutrition, College of Physicians and Surgeons, Columbia University, New York, New York; Stephen Zamenhof, Professor of Microbial Genetics, School of Medicine, University of California at Los Angeles, California.

These reviewers were ably supplemented by the contributions of a long list of advisers, who provided not only counsel and documented information but much needed encouragement as well:

Irving S. Bengelsdorf, Director of Science Communication,

California Institute of Technology, Pasadena, California; R. Quentin Blackwell, Head, Department of Biochemistry, U. S. Naval Medical Research Unit #2, APO San Francisco, California; Roscoe O. Brady, Chief, Development and Metabolic Neurology Branch, National Institute of Neurological Disease and Stroke, National Institutes of Health, Bethesda, Maryland; William F. Brazziel, Professor of Higher Education, University of Connecticut, Storrs, Connecticut; Melvin Calvin, Director of the Laboratory of Chemical Biodynamics, University of California at Berkeley, California; Josué de Castro, President, International Medical Association for the Study of Living Conditions and Health, Neuilly-sur-Seine, France; Bacon F. Chow, Professor of Biochemistry, School of Hygiene and Public Health, Johns Hopkins University, Baltimore, Maryland; Louis K. Diamond, Professor of Pediatrics, School of Medicine, University of California at San Francisco, California; John Dobbing, Professor of Child Health and Pediatrics, University of Manchester, Manchester, England; Philip R. Dodge, Professor of Pediatrics and Neurology and Head, Department of Pediatrics, School of Medicine, Washington University, St. Louis, Missouri; Joseph T. English, President, New York City Health and Hospitals Corporation, New York, New York; Harrington Gosling, Head, Behavioral Science, Faculty of Medicine, University of Dar Es Salaam, Tanzania; Peter D. Gardner, Professor of Chemistry and Dean for Sciences, University of Utah, Salt Lake City, Utah; George G. Graham, Professor of Hygiene and Public Health, Johns Hopkins University, Baltimore, Maryland; Jean Pierre Habicht, Division of Human Development, Instituto de Nutrición de Centro América y Panamá (I.N.C.A.P.), World Health Organization, Guatemala, C.A.; Leonard Herzenberg, Professor of Genetics, School of Medicine, Stanford University, Stanford, California; Frank M. Huennekens, Chairman, Department of Biochemistry, Scripps Clinic and Research Foundation, La Jolla, California; Robert E. Klein, Division of Human Development, Instituto de Nutrición de Centro América y Panamá (I.N.C.A.P.), World Health Organization, Guatemala, C.A.; Abel Lajtha, Director,

New York State Research Institute for Neurochemistry and Drug
Addiction, New York, New York; Robert E. Leakey, Administra-
tive Director, National Museums of Kenya, Nairobi, Kenya;
Joshua Lederberg, Professor and Chairman, Department of
Genetics, School of Medicine, Stanford University, Stanford,
California; Paul Mandel, Director, Institut de Neurochimie, Cen-
tre National de la Recherche Scientifique, Faculté de Médicine,
Université de Strasbourg, France; Jane R. Mercer, Professor of
Sociology, University of California at Riverside, California; John
B. Neilands, Professor of Biochemistry, University of California
at Berkeley, California; Rodolfo Paoletti, Professor, Istituto di
Farmacologia e di Farmacognosia, Università di Milano, Italy;
Colin S. Pittendrigh, Professor of Biological Sciences, Stanford
University, Stanford, California; John K. Pollard, Jr., Vice-
President for Biochemical Development, Calbiochem, San Diego,
California; David Prior, Sanford Greenburger Associates, New
York, New York; Eugene Roberts, Director, Division of Neuro-
sciences, City of Hope National Medical Center, Duarte, Cali-
fornia; Rupert A. L. Perrin, Head, Department of Immunology,
Calbiochem, San Diego, California; Paul D. Saltman, Vice-
Chancellor for Academic Affairs, University of California at San
Diego, California; Richard S. and Marilyn D. Scharffenberg, Lit-
erature Searchers, Riverside, California; Nevin S. Scrimshaw,
Professor and Head, Department of Nutrition and Food Science,
Massachusetts Institute of Technology, Cambridge, Massachu-
setts; Silvio S. Varon, Professor of Biology and Neurosciences,
University of California at San Diego, California; Joseph J.
Vitale, Professor, School of Medicine, Tufts University, Boston,
Massachusetts; Josef Warkany, Professor of Research Pediatrics,
Children's Hospital Medical Center, University of Cincinnati,
Ohio.

I did not always accept advice, counsel, or criticism, and I
alone bear the responsibility for what appears in these pages.

Grateful acknowledgment is made of permission to quote
from the following publications:

Mental Testing, Its History, Principles, and Applications, by

F. L. Goodenough, Rinehart & Company, 1949; "Late 'Catch-up' After Severe Infantile Malnutrition," by G. G. Graham and B. Adrianzen T., *The Johns Hopkins Medical Journal*, 1972; "Nutrition, Growth and Neurointegrative Development: An Experimental and Ecologic Study," by J. Cravioto, E. R. DeLicardie, and H. G. Birch, *Journal of American Academy of Pediatrics*, 1966; *Race and Intelligence, The Fallacies Behind the I.Q. Controversy*, ed. by K. Richardson, D. Spears, and M. Richards, Penguin Books, Ltd., 1972; "Foreign Policy for Disillusioned Liberals," by L. P. Bloomfield, *Foreign Policy*, National Affairs, Inc., 1972; *The Crazy Ape*, by A. Szent-Györgyi, Philosophical Library, 1970; *The Testing of Negro Intelligence*, by A. M. Shuey, Social Science Press, 1966; "Nutrition and Learning. Inadequate Nutrition in Infancy May Result in Permanent Impairment of Mental Function," by H. F. Eichenwald and P. C. Fry, *Science*, American Association for the Advancement of Science, 1969; "The Effects of Intrauterine Malnutrition upon Later Development in Humans," by G. A. Neligan, *Psychiatria, Neurologia, Neurochirurgia*, 1971. The support and publication of this book by Doubleday & Company is an admirable act of faith that was sustained by two talented editors, Elizabeth Knappman and Toni Werbel. They richly deserve my appreciative recognition.

I was fortunate to have ready access to the magnificent library facilities of the University of California at San Diego and the San Diego Public Library. The gracious co-operation of the skilled and attentive staff of these outstanding organizations was invaluable in the preparation of the manuscript. Finally, a personal note of thanks to three remarkable and erudite men who encouraged me to put pen to paper and guided my efforts in the process: Eric Berger, Editor-in-Chief of Scholastic Magazines, Inc., the late Sanford J. Greenburger, and his son Francis, who now heads Sanford J. Greenburger Associates.

ELIE A. SHNEOUR

La Jolla, California
April 1973

Chapter I

THE NATURE OF THE PROBLEM

This is a book about children.

It is written on their behalf because they are unable to express themselves collectively and because they represent the only hope for the future of the human species.

The human brain is most vulnerable to inadequate nutrition during the earliest period of life, and the entire course of human existence is largely determined by the nutrition received during that time. The growth of the human brain during gestation is one of the earliest, most rapid, and most extensive developments of the whole organism. After birth the brain continues to grow at a much faster rate than the rest of the body, so much so that by the time a child is four years old his brain has reached 90 per cent of its adult weight, while the rest of his body has barely made it to the 20 per cent mark.[1]

During this critical period of rapid growth, much more than just an increase in weight is involved. The structure of the brain undergoes profound and complex changes in its anatomy, chemistry, and physiology.[2] Maturation of the brain involves

---

[1] J. A. Harris *et al., The Measurements of Man* (Minneapolis: University of Minnesota Press, 1930).

[2] J. L. Conel, *The Postnatal Development of the Human Cortex* (Cambridge: Harvard University Press, 1963).

the manufacture of substances in amounts sufficient not only for the growth of the brain but also for its normal operation.[3] Without adequate nutrition, a concept of great complexity in itself, the systematic now-or-never schedule of brain development is affected. Deficiencies now can never be made up later.[4]

Unequivocal direct evidence is lacking, and a great deal of information is still needed, before the relationship among early-life diet, brain development, and mental abilities can be confirmed. But there is an already vast and rapidly growing body of data that support the concept that native intelligence can be permanently impaired by inadequate diet.[5,6] We cannot wait until all the evidence is available in complete detail before action is taken to alleviate existing malnutrition; many of its consequences are already clear-cut and serious enough to warrant immediate attention.

In many ways this problem has much in common with the consequences of human exposure to radioactivity. The long-term effects of early-life malnutrition as well as the effects of radiation become manifest long after exposure, when it is too late to apply effective remedies. There is still much controversy about the exact nature and extent of radiation damage, but there is no question that such damage does occur and that it has an irremediable component. Similarly, the exact nature and extent of irreversible brain damage resulting from early-life malnutrition is not known, but such an outcome is not only possible but probable enough to deserve serious consideration now.

The scope of the problem is worldwide. More than 350 million children, seven out of every ten under the age of six, 20 million of them in the United States alone, suffer from the effects of mal-

---

[3] W. A. Himwich, *International Review of Neurobiology* 4 (1962), p. 117.
[4] J. P. Scott, "Critical Periods," *Society for Research in Child Development Monograph 28* (1963), p. 1.
[5] J. Bowlby, "Critical Phases in the Development of Social Responses in Man and Other Animals," *Prospects in Psychiatric Research*, ed. by J. M. Tanner (Oxford: Blackwell Scientific Publications, 1952).
[6] H. F. Eichenwald and P. C. Fry, "Nutrition and Learning," *Science* 163 (1969), pp. 644–48.

nutrition or starvation. At least half of the world's population has survived a period of severe deprivation during childhood.[7]

In the United States hunger is much more widespread than most people believe, but the evidence for it is overwhelming.[8] It is the children of the poor, those who have failed to receive a diet adequate for normal brain development, who may be condemned to a substandard level of intelligence, unable to compete effectively for survival and a meaningful life for themselves and their progeny. In this country it means members of some of our largest minorities, people in decaying cities, on welfare rolls and in overcrowded jails.

Yet this crucial issue has not received the attention of politicians, even though it has been recognized for a long time by scientific workers in the field.[9]

While biomedical scientists are not blameless for this serious impasse, the major responsibility must rest with those who determine priorities at the highest policy-making levels of government. The skyrocketing cost of welfare support, crime and police protection, judicial proceedings, and hospital or penal custody is many times that of prevention. To treat rather than to prevent is a choice made by most governing institutions, both public and private. Medical insurance payments in the United States are based on treatment after a disease has developed; almost no provision exists for payment to prevent the disease from developing. The lack of imagination and leadership exhibited by our insuring institutions in this regard is beyond the ken of rational men. Their folly, however, is exceeded only by the choice of priorities made by national leaders.

The nations of the world, but primarily the U.S.A. and the

---

[7] M. Winick, "Malnutrition and Brain Development," *Journal of Pediatrics* 74 (1969), p. 667.

[8] *Nutrition and Human Needs,* Hearings before U. S. Senate Select Committee on Nutrition and Human Needs, 1968–71 (Washington: U. S. Government Printing Office, 1969–71).

[9] I. N. Kugelmass, L. E. Poull, and E. L. Samuel, "Nutritional Improvement of Child Mentality," *American Journal of Medical Science* 208 (1944), p. 631.

U.S.S.R., have spent since the end of World War II *more than four thousand billion dollars* for armaments. Great powers and underdeveloped nations alike have spent inordinate portions of their resources for waging wars justified in the interests of self-betterment, while they have ignored the problems whose solution is necessary to improve the human condition.

Malnutrition, poverty, and starvation are related problems whose significant alleviation is possible within one generation. The means exist to achieve this goal, if only massive organized resources can be made available with the necessary sustained effort and motivation.

In the words of the biologist Albert Szent-Györgyi, discoverer of vitamin C and Nobel laureate, "Why does man behave like a perfect idiot? . . . Today is the first time in man's history that he is able to truly enjoy life, free of cold, hunger and disease. It is the first time he is able to satisfy all his basic needs. Conversely, it is also the first time in his history that man has the capability of exterminating himself in one blow or making his tragically shrinking, lovely little globe uninhabitable by pollution or over-population. One would expect that any idiot could make a wise choice between these two alternatives. . . ."[10]

By the year 2000, today's world population will have doubled to 7.4 billion, requiring those persons able to work to support, mainly through taxation, an increasing number of mentally and physiologically crippled human beings. The world's population is adding the equivalent of a city of two hundred thousand persons every twenty-four hours, and more than half of the children born will suffer the crippling effects of malnutrition in the first critical years of their existence.

Political awareness of poverty in the United States arrived with the civil rights movement. In April 1967, Senators Robert Kennedy of New York and Joseph Clark of Pennsylvania visited small towns in the Mississippi delta. They saw a level of raw hunger and poverty unequaled by the worst conditions the black

---

[10] A. Szent-Györgyi, *The Crazy Ape* (New York: Philosophical Library, 1970), p. 11. Quoted by permission.

South had experienced during the depression of the 1930s. Senator Kennedy, usually a master of self-control, was shocked speechless by what he saw. He mumbled to an aide that he had seen bad things in West Virginia, but never had he seen anything like this anywhere in the United States.[11]

A team of noted pediatricians followed the senators to Mississippi in May 1967. Their testimony before a Congressional subcommittee on July 11 and 12 of that year makes disturbing reading and shows little evidence of any humanity for the children involved. ". . . In boys and girls in every county we visited, [we saw] obvious evidence of severe malnutrition, with injury to the body's tissues—its muscles, bones, and skin as well as an associated psychological state of fatigue, listlessness, and exhaustion. . . . We saw homes with children who are lucky to eat one meal a day—and that one inadequate so far as vitamins, minerals or protein is concerned. We saw children who don't get to drink milk, don't get to eat fruit, green vegetables, or meat. They live on starches—grits, bread, Kool-Aid. . . . Not only are these children receiving no food from the government, they are also getting no medical attention whatsoever. They are out of sight and ignored. They are living under such primitive conditions that we found it hard to believe we were examining American children of the twentieth century. . . ."[12]

These words are echoed by others who describe a situation not limited to any one part of the country. Grossly inadequate nutrition for poor children, even when countered with a multiplicity of welfare programs, is the rule rather than the exception.

Dr. Aaron Altshul, Special Assistant for Nutrition Improvement, U. S. Department of Agriculture, has stated: "It is a common observation that the children of the 30 million poverty-

11 "Clark and Kennedy Visit the Poor of Mississippi," New York Times, April 12, 1967, p. 29.
12 Hunger and Malnutrition in America, Hearings before Subcommittee on Employment, Manpower and Poverty of the Committee on Labor and Public Welfare, U. S. Senate, 90th Congress, 1st session, July 1967. (Washington: U. S. Government Printing Office, 1967), p. 46.

stricken people in the United States may get enough food through welfare programs. But do they get enough proteins? Mostly they eat starchy foods—potatoes, grits, cornpone, bread, beans and so forth. If the family has meat, cheese, nuts or fish, it goes mostly to adults. So children suffer brain damage that is never overcome, irrespective of the amounts of protein consumed later. These children, being deprived of normal brain development, do not do well in school. They do not have the intelligence, the initiative or the motivation that stem from normal brain capacity."[13]

Malnourished pregnant women give birth to a significantly larger number of premature infants. These children have a much higher mortality rate than those who are delivered at term. Those who survive are much more likely to exhibit evidence of brain damage. This was the burden of the testimony given by Dr. Charles Upton Lowe, Scientific Director of the National Institute of Child Health and Human Welfare, before the Senate Select Committee on Nutrition and Human Needs, chaired by Senator George S. McGovern of South Dakota. Dr. Lowe said: "The earlier malnutrition exists, the more devastatingly it impinges on growth and development. . . . When an infant undergoes severe nutritional deprivation during the first months of life, his brain fails to synthesize protein and cells at normal rates and consequently suffers a decrease as great as 20 percent in the cell number. . . . When very small at birth, as many as 50 percent of the prematurely born infants grow to maturity with an intellectual competence significantly below that which would be expected when compared with siblings and even with age peers. . . . The rate of premature births is far higher, in some cases two and three times higher [in families living in poverty] than it is in more well-to-do families. Finally, the prevalence of intellectual compromise and even mental deficiency may be from three to five times as frequent in children of families living in poverty. In effect, malnutrition, high infant mortality and prematurity rates

---

[13] Quoted in W. Johnson, "Protein and Poverty, or School Lunches Are Too Late," *Child Welfare*, June 1967.

and high levels of mental deficiencies coexist as a constellation of abnormalities that are most frequent among our families living in poverty. . . ."[14]

In this country, major biomedical efforts have pinpointed a number of fatal diseases for eradication, including poliomyelitis, cancer, and cardiovascular disorders. There has been a particular emphasis on diseases that affect children, and the news media often report cases that elicit immediate and generous response from individuals and organizations. But the oldest and most persistent scourge of mankind, which most often affects children and destroys their life opportunities—the triad of hunger, poverty, and ignorance—is largely forgotten by the community.

Yet the child crippled by defective mental capacities is just as damaged as if he were the victim of polio. Society has made iron lungs and wheelchairs available to the polio victim, but has nothing to offer the child who cannot learn, nor later his own children, who will suffer because of his inability to earn a living. Thus not only the child but also his progeny will suffer from the crippling effects of hunger.[15] From this vicious circle there can be no escape without the understanding leadership and action of government supported by an informed electorate.

Despite the evidence presented to the U. S. Congress since 1967, and in particular the expert testimony given before the U. S. Senate Select Committee on Nutrition and Human Needs, the problem of hunger in the U.S.A. has still not surfaced as a major political issue. There has been much political rhetoric on the subject, but no action remotely commensurate with the magnitude of the problem. A skeptical public still does not understand the significance of this human and economic problem for which each person in this country pays an enormous forfeit.

---

14 *Nutrition and Human Needs,* Hearings before U. S. Senate Select Committee on Nutrition and Human Needs, Part 3, "The National Nutrition Survey," January 1969 (Washington: U. S. Government Printing Office, 1969), pp. 1082–1104.
15 *Hunger Causes Mental Retardation,* A Report to the California State Assembly Committee on Health and Welfare, October 31, 1969.

Those who have seen what hunger really means are not likely ever to forget it. And those who have experienced it personally, such as the surviving victims of the concentration camps of World War II, have known lasting effects that have changed the course of their lives.[16] Whereas the victims of hunger often look healthy and well-fed, this appearance is deceiving and is caused by the swelling of tissues, a common symptom of sustained poor nutrition in children. The ignorance of this fact may help explain Mississippi Governor Paul Johnson's callous response to a reporter's question about hunger among the black poor in Mississippi: "All the Negroes I've seen around here are so fat they shine!"[17]

The human brain is by far the most complicated organ of the body, composed of precisely interrelated parts that can be affected in subtle ways. Mild but sustained malnutrition (often called hidden or occult malnutrition) during the early, critical period of life may cause damage to the brain just as readily as will outright starvation, but the results will be more difficult to identify.

The degree of mental deficiency appears to be related to the age of the victim and the severity and duration of poor nutrition. This insidious damage often becomes painfully evident only when the child is confronted by a group learning situation in school. Dr. David Coursin, Director of Research of the Research Institute, St. Joseph Hospital, Lancaster, Pennsylvania, has summarized the results of studies of chronically undernourished school children primarily in Mexico and Costa Rica, two countries that have well-established educational systems with good, available school records. Even when these children were systematically fed an adequate diet for several months, their school performance did not catch up to the normal average level of school performance. The children exhibited deficiencies of between 10

---

[16] L. Eitinger, "Concentration Camp Survivors in Norway and Israel," *Israel Journal of Medical Sciences* 1 (1965), pp. 883–97. This report has a bibliography consisting of seventeen other pertinent references.

[17] N. Kotz, *Let Them Eat Promises* (New York: Anchor Books, 1971), p. 36.

and 25 per cent, depending upon how young they were when they experienced deprivation and on how long it lasted.[18]

Relating early nutritional deficiencies to subsequent mental dysfunctions is difficult because of the problem of making clear-cut observations. Rats, for example, have been used for years in psychological experiments in which they run through mazes of varying complexity to find their food reward or escape an electric shock. One can surgically remove as much as half of a rat brain before his performance in a simple maze is affected. In fact, one can hardly tell the difference between a normal and an operated rat in such simple mazes. But if these rats are put through increasingly complicated mazes, the difference between a normal and an operated rat becomes readily evident. In very complex mazes small differences in brain surgery show up very clearly.

Such experiments cannot be done with human beings, and clear-cut answers for humans thus become more difficult to obtain. But translated into human terms the above experiments suggest that the effects of brain damage may not become apparent until the victims are compelled to use increasingly advanced mental skills to survive.

By accidents of history, sustained by contempt and neglect, it is mainly the non-white minorities of this nation that have been the victims of inadequate early-life diet. Poverty and its direct attendant consequences show up clearly in infant-mortality statistics. The non-white infants of less than one year of age, U.S. Census figures show, are dying at nearly twice the rate of the white infants. The white infants have shown a slowly decreasing death rate, due mainly to the benefits of good economic conditions and medical services, while the non-white infant death rate has been steadily increasing.

The same kind of dismal picture has emerged from comparisons of the intellectual performance of white and non-white children, most of which has been ascribed to inherited rather than

---

[18] D. B. Coursin, "Undernutrition and Brain Function," *Borden's Review of Nutrition Research* 26 (1965), p. 3.

acquired factors. This belief of long standing was given strong impetus in 1958 by the publication of a book by Dr. Audrey M. Shuey, Professor of Psychology at Randolph-Macon Woman's College, Lynchburg, Virginia, entitled *The Testing of Negro Intelligence.* In the introduction, the author wrote: "It is not the purpose of this book to prove that Negroes are socially, morally, or intellectually inferior to whites; nor is its purpose to demonstrate that Negroes are the equal of or are superior to whites in these several characteristics. Rather, it is the intention of the writer to convey with some degree of clarity and order the results of many years of research on one aspect of Negro behavior and to assess objectively the ever-growing literature on this subject."[19]

This 578-page book is a detailed study of the mental status of blacks in the United States based on intelligence tests of large numbers of persons over a period of fifty years. In samplings among preschool, school, and college students, enlisted men and officers, transients, delinquents, criminals, gifted and mentally deficient individuals, and in comparisons among high-status whites and Negroes, rural and urban dwellers in the southern, border, and northern states, Dr. Shuey found remarkably consistent differences between whites and blacks, in which the blacks demonstrated relatively poorer performance than the whites. The dubious conclusion was that, taken together, these data pointed inevitably to the existence of a native, that is to say inherited, difference between Negroes and whites as determined by intelligence tests.

In early 1965 Assistant Secretary of Labor Daniel P. Moynihan wrote a confidential report for President Lyndon B. Johnson that became public knowledge only after the Watts riots in Los Angeles that summer. That report suggested that the bitter legacy of slavery and the resulting matriarchal structure of the American black family placed the black at a significant competi-

---

[19] A. M. Shuey, *The Testing of Negro Intelligence*, 2nd ed. (New York: Social Science Press, 1966), p. 1. Quoted by permission.

tive disadvantage in the white, predominantly patriarchal, society.

A year later Dr. James S. Coleman, Department of Sociology, Johns Hopkins University, published the report of a major study of some four thousand U.S. public schools and their more than six hundred thousand students. An essential message conveyed by the Coleman Report was that black students showed consistently poorer scholastic achievement than white students at every grade level. As the students progressed from the first to the twelfth grades, these differences became increasingly marked. While the Coleman Report recognized the effects of segregation and racist social customs on these results, it noted that the removal of these impediments did not seem to greatly affect the outcome of the findings.[20]

The growing controversy was fueled by the publication, in 1969, of a persuasive analysis of the problem by Dr. Arthur R. Jensen, Professor of Educational Psychology at the University of California at Berkeley.[21] Dr. Jensen's response to this rhetorical question was that hereditary differences in inborn mental ability are not susceptible to significant improvement, no matter how dedicated an effort might be made to overcome such differences.

With the publication of Dr. Jensen's paper, even though it had been written for academic colleagues and couched in lucid but technical terms, the controversy became public. The editors of the *Harvard Education Review* cautiously reprinted the paper in a book compiling the pro-and-con discussions that raged through the subsequent issues of this journal among Dr. Jensen's peers.[22] They included such titles as "Inadequate Evidence and Illogical Conclusions" (by Dr. Jerome S. Kagan, Department of Developmental Psychology, Harvard University), "Has Com-

---

[20] J. S. Coleman *et al., Equality of Educational Opportunity*, U. S. Department of Health, Education and Welfare, 1966.
[21] A. R. Jensen, "How Much Can We Boost I.Q. and Scholastic Achievement?" *Harvard Educational Review* 39 (1969).
[22] *Environment, Heredity and Intelligence*, Reprint Series No. 2 (Cambridge, Mass.: Harvard University Graduate School of Education, 1969).

pensatory Education Failed? Has It Been Attempted?" (by Dr.
J. McV. Hunt, Department of Psychology and Education, University of Illinois, and former Director of the Coordination Center, National Laboratory of Early Childhood Education).

The controversy became considerably more heated when
otherwise responsible writers such as Dr. Hans J. Eysenck,
Director, Institute of Psychiatry, Maudsley Hospital, London,
jumped into the fray.[23] Dr. Eysenck argued in support of the by
now emotionally explosive postulate, based on complex technical
arguments yet to be demonstrated, that intelligence as measured
by I.Q. (intelligence quotient) tests is 80 per cent inherited
and only 20 per cent acquired through environmental influences.
While the text is guarded, the author's bias is obvious. Blacks are
likely to have, on the whole, intelligence inferior to that of
whites, writes Dr. Eysenck.

This conclusion was supported, in part, by the anecdotal thesis
that the American Negro is intellectually inferior because of the
negative selection process introduced by slavery. White slave
traders wanted dull beasts of burden, this argument goes, which
put intelligence at a strong disadvantage. In addition to which,
this argument continues, the bright ones were smart enough to
get away. This simplistic "explanation" and others like it had
been laid to rest in 1941, when Dr. Melville J. Herskovits, a noted
anthropologist and Director of the Program of African Studies,
Northwestern University, published a comprehensive study for
the Carnegie Corporation of New York.[24]

Another notable effort, that of Professor Richard Herrnstein
of Harvard University, led to a riot[25] at the Boston editorial offices
of the magazine. While the tone of this article was restrained,
Dr. Herrnstein's conclusion was the same; i.e., hereditary differences as measured by I.Q. tests are real and might as well be

---

[23] H. J. Eysenck, *The I.Q. Argument: Race, Intelligence and Education*
(Freeport, N.Y.: Library Press, 1971).
[24] M. J. Herskovits, *The Myth of the Negro Past* (Boston: Beacon Press,
1958). (Original edition New York: Harper & Brothers, 1941).
[25] R. Herrnstein, "I.Q.," *Atlantic Monthly*, September 1971, pp. 43–64.

accepted as fact, since social standing and structure are largely determined by them. The reader will note in a later chapter that I.Q. scores, intelligence, and mental ability are not synonymous, and that serious reservations exist in the interpretation of these terms.

As if this were not enough, Dr. William B. Shockley, Department of Engineering Science, Stanford University, coinventor of the transistor and Nobel laureate, had since 1965 been adding the weight of his scientific reputation to his unsuccessful insistence that the august National Academy of Sciences, an organization chartered by the U. S. Congress, sponsor research to resolve this problem once and for all. As the reader of this book will appreciate, this type of research is easier said than done, if indeed it can be done at all.

That there are hereditary differences among human beings is an undeniable fact. That we are all, individually and collectively, the product of our genetic heritage is equally certain. *But there exists no evidence strong enough to sustain the argument that mental ability might be the favored province of any one human group.* Before any concept involving relative genetic mental potential can be made a legitimate subject of investigation, the many layers of environmental influences will have to be systematically stripped away in quantitative terms. The day when this can be done lies well in the future.

It is not the purpose of this book to join this polemical conflict but rather to attempt a reasoned and documented analysis of the issue, in which the damaging effect of early-life malnutrition on mental development may be a critical factor. This has not been done by any of the leading participants in the controversy. Our purpose is to plant a seed of doubt among those whose minds may be closing prematurely on an evolving issue. While a solution to the early-life malnutrition problem will not resolve the whole issue of mental deficiency, underprivilege, and poverty, it is a required first step, without which every other effort is likely to be meaningless and futile.

Genetics, nutrition, disease, family and school stimulation, and

other environmental effects both subtle and obvious all interact
to affect mental capacity. How does one distinguish among them?
Is it easier to identify nutritional effects than genetic factors, and
if so how does one go about it?

The clearest possible answer is that among all *early* environmental influences, that of nutrition is by far the most important
and significant factor. Proper nutrition will not salvage a severely
deficient hereditary makeup, but the vast majority of human
beings who survive do not a priori belong to this category. Their
pedigree gives them a level of mental ability at least adequate
to the tasks they must perform to prosper as human beings in a
competitive social environment.

The reverse side of this coin is equally compelling. The acceptance of the postulate that some human groups are intellectually
inferior to others carries with it extremely serious potential consequences for all of mankind. Given the importance of this matter, one must have an absolute certitude that it is in fact a correct
conclusion.

We do not have this assurance now.[26]

We are not likely to have it in the foreseeable future.

We must therefore seek to identify those controllable early
factors which are known to damage the most precious of man's
biological equipment, and act to eliminate them. If we are the
civilized people we claim to be, we will recognize no other alternative.

Major elements of the relationship between nutrition and brain
development are discussed in the following chapters.

We begin with the story of the human brain.

---

[26] The author is indebted for this strong and lucid statement to Professor
Paul Mandel, Director of the Neurochemistry Institute, University of Strasbourg, France: "L'acceptance du postulat de l'infériorité raciale conduit à
des conséquences extrèmement sérieuses. Devant l'importance de la chose
il faut en avoir la certitude absolue que c'est vrai. Or, nous ne l'avons pas."

Chapter II

THE HUMAN BRAIN

The human brain is the culmination of almost 3 billion years of evolutionary history. It reflects the highest degree of biological development achieved by any living thing. The most complex structure in creation, it is the site of man's supremacy in the animal kingdom. It is the organ that allows him to dominate his environment and control his destiny.

The earliest known living cells appeared in the primitive oceans of the planet earth more than 2.7 billion years ago, and their remains have been found in Precambrian rocks of what is now Africa.[1] These cells, probably similar to today's blue green algae, were completely passive organisms, unable to respond to changes in the environment. Their survival and reproduction depended upon the maintenance of a favorable supply of energy from sunlight and food from the oceans. These tropical waters then still contained an accumulation of foodstuffs left over from an earlier period, during which the first organic matter was formed on the primitive earth,[2] described by the English biologist J. B. S. Haldane as "a hot thin soup."

---

[1] A. Holmes, "The Oldest Dated Minerals of the Rhodesian Shield," *Nature* 173 (1954), p. 612.
[2] S. L. Miller and H. C. Urey, "Organic Compound Synthesis on the Primitive Earth," *Science* 130 (1959), p. 245.

Under these mild conditions the cells floating in the waters proliferated, and competition for food and light began in earnest. These independent cells did not have a nervous system, let alone a brain. But some of them acquired, by random mutation, the ability to identify food and light and, most importantly, to respond to these stimuli by swimming into the areas of their greatest abundance. This evolutionary change gave the cells that had acquired it an enormous competitive advantage over cells not so endowed. The eventual result of this struggle for survival was the disappearance of the more primitive cells as they were swamped by a greatly increased number and diversity of the more advanced ones.

Thus response to the environment was a vital aspect of evolution, of which the eventual development of the human brain is the ultimate expression. Evolution by natural selection is one of the greatest conceptions of modern man, ranking with Einstein's special theory of relativity. It is certainly the most important concept in biology, in which the brain plays a major role. Like all brilliant insights, Darwin's theory of evolution by natural selection is based on simple propositions: (1) progeny outnumber their parents; (2) in spite of this high fecundity the total population remains relatively stable because of limitation of space and available resources; and (3) the abundant progeny are endowed with a much greater diversity of traits than are their parents. Charles Darwin's deduction from these simple premises was that there was in nature a continuous struggle for existence, and that only those best fitted to their environment would survive and reproduce their kind, while those with unfavorable attributes would be eliminated.

A remarkable and well-documented example of natural selection occurred in the mid-1800s, during England's industrial expansion.[3] Most of the moths in the countryside were light-colored, but scientific observers of the time noted that the light-colored moths were gradually being replaced by dark ones until

---

[3] H. B. D. Kettlewell, "The Phenomenon of Industrial Melanism in Lepidoptera," *Annual Reviews of Entomology* 6 (1962), pp. 245–62.

as many as 90 per cent of them in the industrial areas were dark. This puzzling phenomenon was eventually explained as follows: While the country remained rural, the light-colored moths matched well the color of the tree trunks, while the dark moths stood out and easily fell prey to hungry birds. As the soot from coal-burning factories gradually darkened the trees, the situation was reversed, i.e., the light-colored moths now stood out and were early and frequent victims of bird predators, while the dark moths now were able to blend with their surroundings and thus survive and reproduce their kind in increasing numbers over their light counterparts.

Evolution did not proceed gradually and inexorably in one, preordained direction. Chance played a dominant role, and diversity insured that at least some cells possessed traits that would be advantageous in the existing environment. The environment itself, of course, changed also. Some advantages in one circumstance could prove disastrous in another.

By trial and error, by modifications that appeared and then disappeared when they proved to be evolutionary dead ends, and by random, lucky, and timely appearance of attributes that were favorably matched by environmental changes, did evolution go forward. The development of a nervous system proved to be perhaps the most radical improvement that a group of cells could achieve for its collective survival and prosperity. This occurred early in the geological history of the planet.

Single cells evolved to form clusters of cells able to interact with each other and to specialize. Some members of the clusters became proficient at gathering food, others at digesting it, while still others connected themselves into a net capable of identifying and transmitting information about the environment throughout the colony. This was the beginning of the development of a true nervous system—a primitive nerve net, to be sure, but effective enough to recognize both opportunity and danger.

We still find on the shores of seas and oceans descendants of these early animals. They belong to the phylum known as the coelenterates, which includes the hydra, the jellyfish, and the sea anemone.

The nerve net was only the first step up the evolutionary ladder in the developing nervous system. It provided the organism with the simplest possible mechanism for gathering information about basic environmental variables. But the response of such an organism to a stimulus was very slow and uncoordinated (as anyone who has ever touched a sea anemone and watched it close on his finger can testify), because there was no central direction of the functions of the neural net. The acquisition of a neural center, called *cephalization*, was the process by which a brain eventually emerged.

An interesting modern example of this developmental stage of the nervous system is found in the flatworm planaria. It has a head, with a very primitive brain and simple light-sensitive spots that could be called eyes. Because the planaria has eyes and other sense organs and because information about the outside world can be conveyed by these sense organs to the brain, this little flatworm can respond more quickly to what goes on around it, can move about more rapidly, and can do much more as a living organism than can the jellyfish. But the flatworm brain is very limited; it cannot coordinate movement. In fact, one can surgically remove the planaria's brain, and the flatworm will still be able to move around as if nothing had happened, except for the loss of sensory response to the environment.

Coordination of movement by the brain is such a complex function that apparently the brain could not achieve it at this point in evolution without help from the peripheral nerve net. This became possible with segmentation of the organism into separate parts able to handle local problems without reference to the brain. Only when it was necessary to take concerted action could the brain override local intersegmental reflexes and coordinate a mass response by the whole organism. Such is the case, for instance, with the earthworm. And anyone who has ever observed an earthworm, or sacrificed part of one to a fishing hook, will recognize that earthworm segments seem to have a life of their own, in addition to an integral one possessed by the whole animal controlled by its brain.

This segmentation is found in a much more elaborate form in man. The human nerve net consists of nerve fibers that issue from the spinal cord, between the vertebrae, and radiate to specific areas of the human body. Thus man can in effect be sliced into some thirty-three segments, most of which can handle simple reflex actions (such as jerking a hand away from a hot stove without direct and immediate action of the brain) but which are connected with and coordinated by the brain.

The geology of the earth began with the formation of the earth's crust about 4.6 billion years ago. The first 4 billion years have left very little in the way of a fossil record. This long and dimly perceived era is known as the Precambrian. Beginning with the Paleozoic era, which started about 600 million years ago, abundant fossil records exist, and most of the stages of evolution described up to this point took place during the early part of the Paleozoic era.

About 500 million years ago there appeared a group of animals whose likes had never been seen before on the earth. Although these animals were quite different from their ancestors, they nevertheless retained such successful features as cephalization and segmentation of their nervous systems. The most significant feature they possessed, however, at least during a part of their life, was a hollow, cartilaginous backbone, which ran from top to bottom along the back, the *notochord*. A few of these animals, of which the contemporary primitive fish amphioxus is a leading example, retained the notochord throughout life. But most of the others gradually substituted for the notochord a series of vertebrae. The vertebrates are unique in that they possess an internal skeleton, articulated at the spine and protecting the central nervous system, surmounted by the brain, which is in turn protected by the skull. A rigid structure confers the mechanical advantages of rapid motion and greatly increased animal size, as well as the less obvious advantage of safety. The skull provided a secure housing for the brain and its associated major sense organs of vision, sound, and smell. Protected from the environment, these organs were able to develop more rapidly and with much greater sophistication than those of other living organisms. The notochord, therefore, proved to be a quantum jump in evolution. It made possible high mental capabilities, including intelligence.

The predominant subphylum of the vertebrates includes the fishes, reptiles, birds, and mammals, of which man is the most highly advanced example. Because of their brain and central nervous system, the vertebrates are immeasurably more efficient and responsive to the environment than any other living thing. They literally took over the earth in succession: first the fishes, then the reptiles, the mammals, and finally modern man.

The Paleozoic era lasted until 225 million years ago and ushered in the Mesozoic era, which lasted for more than 150 million years. The Mesozoic was the age during which the great reptiles, the dinosaurs, the largest animals in geological history, roamed the earth. An example was the 65-foot-long *Brontosaurus*. This great reptile was controlled by an amazingly minuscule, one-pound brain surmounting its 35-ton bulk (see Table I).

Almost unnoticed, there appeared during that time an increasing number of small, warm-blooded, furtive, and inconspicuous mouse-like animals. The dinosaurs from their august fleshy pedestals did not seem to care; they all but ignored these swift-moving, relatively intelligent creatures that arose from the reptiles themselves and started the long line of mammals (Latin, *mammae:* breasts). Their brain was orders of magnitude more advanced than that of the dinosaurs. One of the main reasons for this advantage was that the most successful among them were placental; that is, they carried their young within the mother's body, protected from the environment during a long and laborious growing period, which allowed for extensive development, and they were fed from milk-secreting mammary glands after birth during the remainder of this process. Thus their brain could reach potentials beyond anything that had ever been possible before.

About 75 million years ago, after the longest reign of any group of animals on earth, the dinosaurs disappeared, with a suddenness that has still not been satisfactorily explained. But it seems likely that their inadequate brain must have played a significant, if not a major, role in their swift decline, as the data in Table I suggest.

TABLE I

RATIO OF BRAIN WEIGHT TO TOTAL WEIGHT[4]

Brontosaurus	1/100,000
Crocodile	1/5,000
Elephant	1/600
Gorilla	1/200
Man	1/45
Mouse	1/40
Porpoise	1/38
Marmoset	1/19
Squirrel monkey	1/12

Thus, with increasing variety and sophistication of functions, the brains of the vertebrate animals reflected these changes by striking increases in both proportion and size.

The disappearance of the dinosaurs coincided with significant climatic changes and with the beginning of the modern era, the Cenozoic. As the dinosaurs left a competitive void, the population of mammals literally exploded both in numbers and in kind.

The climate of the earth during the early years of the Cenozoic era was warm, humid, and milder than it is today. Palm trees were growing on the site of what is now London, and in the United States these trees could be found as far north as the Canadian border. It was the golden age of mammalian diversification into the many orders that are the immediate ancestors of the vertebrate animals of today. One of these orders, the primates (Latin, *primus:* first) had acquired, through evolution, two extraordinary advantages, which laid the basis for the eventual

[4] Adapted from S. Cobb, "Brain Size," *Archives of Neurology* 12 (1965), pp. 555–61.

dominance of man and his technology. These were the opposable thumb, which made it possible for these animals to grasp objects, and stereoscopic vision. The eyes of other animals are found on opposite sides of the head, and their vision covers separate fields of view.

The achievement of stereoscopic vision required that the eyes migrate to the front of a flattened face, so that the sight of one eye would overlap that of the other. Stereoscopic vision allowed the accurate judgment of object size and distance. Coupled with hands skilled at grasping, these sensational attributes allowed rapid and safe movement from branch to branch, avoiding ground-based predators. This endowment permitted the primates to pick fruits and to catch swift-moving insects for food. The co-ordination of sight with manipulation also gave them the ability to make and use tools and weapons and to engage in hunting. A dramatic and sustained increase in brain size, complexity, and competence took place simultaneously with the development of these skills and gave effect to these evolutionary manipulative and visual advantages.

In one of the best analyses of brain evolution to date, Dr. Philip Tobias of Columbia University graphically demonstrated that increasing brain size is the most striking sustained trend shown in the hominid (family of man and his ancestors) fossil record. A larger brain, the most evident hallmark of that evolution, must have conferred a clear advantage, and down through the ages this attribute must have afforded greater opportunities for survival than did a smaller brain.[5]

These advantages were to have very great survival value, because soon afterward the primates were subjected to drastic changes in climate. These changes were heralded by one of the most geologically disturbed periods of the earth's history, involving violent volcanic activity and extensive mountain-building, which changed the face of continents. The vast lava beds of the Columbia Plateau in the northwest United States, the Alps, the

---

[5] P. V. Tobias, *The Brain in Hominid Evolution* (New York: Columbia University Press, 1971), p. 114.

Caucasus, and the Coast Range of California are testimony to these gigantic upheavals, some of which continue to this day.

Concurrent with these events, the climate grew progressively colder, signaling the coming of the first of several ice ages, about 2 million years ago. Surprisingly, however, these great periods of widespread glaciation do not appear to have caused the extinction of many animals or plants, but did result in a rapid redistribution of living things over the surface of the planet. Some large mammals such as the mammoth, the mastodon, the ground sloth, and the magnificent saber-toothed tiger, did become extinct, but it seems more likely that their disappearance was the result of hunting by early man.[6] Evidently, as soon as he appeared on earth, ancestral man's ability to play havoc with his environment was already manifest. Most important, however, is the fact that the ice age saw an extraordinarily rapid advance in the evolution of the hominid primates (see Figure 1).

As the earth's climate cooled, the early hominid *Ramapithecus,* the oldest fossil man known (whose remains amount to only pieces of a jaw) roamed the remaining tropical areas now known as India and Africa. *Ramapithecus* gave way to *Australopithecus,* whose remains have been found in widely scattered parts of the world, suggesting a very wide distribution. *Australopithecus* was a biped of small stature, with a brain only one third the size of that of modern man. *Australopithecus* was followed by a number of increasingly larger and more man-like primates with many confusing names and descriptions; actually, the main sequence is simple and well established.[7]

The several hominids recognized by anthropologists overlapped each other, so they were often found to be contemporary for a period of time. *Australopithecus* was the ancestor of *Homo erectus,* and like him was a ground dweller and a fashioner and user of progressively more sophisticated stone tools. *Homo erectus* probably lived between two hundred thousand and seven

---

[6] A. L. McAlester, *The History of Life* (Englewood Cliffs, N.J.: Prentice-Hall, Inc., 1968), p. 127.
[7] Ibid., p. 139.

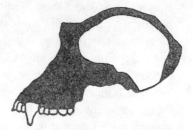

ANTHROPOID APE.
chimpanzee

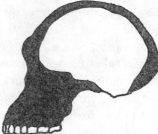

AUSTRALOPITHECUS
500,000 to 2 million years ago

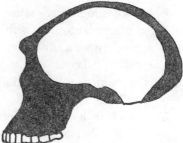

HOMO ERECTUS
200,000 to 700,000 years ago

Figure 1
Major steps in hominid evolution
A modern anthropoid ape skull silhouette is shown for comparison.
Note the size of the cranial cavities and the slant of the face silhouettes.

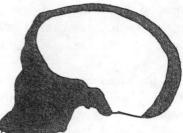

NEANDERTHAL MAN
35,000 to 100,000 years ago

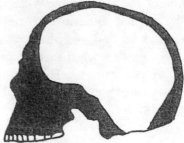

CRO-MAGNON MAN
10,000 to 35,000 years ago

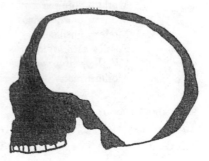

MODERN MAN
european

hundred thousand years ago. His descendants belong to the genus *Homo sapiens*, of which "Neanderthal man", clearly a member of the family of modern man, is the best-known early example.

It has often been stated that since early members of the hominid family had the appearance of apes, Darwin's theory of evolution meant that man must be descended from monkeys. This is not true. While at first glance it might have been difficult to tell *Australopithecus* from a contemporary ape, since both could walk on two feet in an upright position and had opposable thumbs and stereoscopic vision, they nevertheless differed in one striking and fundamental respect: *Australopithecus* and his descendants had overwhelmingly larger brains and overridingly higher intelligence than the apes that were contemporary with them (see Figure 1). The hominids kept pace with these developments and stayed continuously ahead of the apes, as Table II demonstrates.

TABLE II
AVERAGE CRANIAL CAPACITY[8]

Modern chimpanzee	394 cc.
Modern orangutan	411 cc.
Modern gorilla	506 cc.
Fossil *Australopithecus*	494 cc.
Fossil *Homo erectus*	935 cc.
Modern man	1,400 cc.

The most recent genus of man, *Homo sapiens* (Latin, *homo:* man; *sapiens:* wise) is only a few thousand years old, having appeared during the last glacial age. His kind is found in great variety all over the world, with differences in skin color, stature, and temperament. But this great diversity arose from the same ancestral stock and shares many more common features than

[8] Cranial capacity must be distinguished from brain volume, which is smaller, but it is a meaningful approximation of brain size. Adapted from P. V. Tobias, *The Brain in Hominid Evolution* (New York: Columbia University Press, 1971), p. 30.

differences. Among these shared features is the anatomy of the brain itself. The average adult brain weighs approximately 1,400 grams (3 pounds) and represents about 2 per cent of the total body weight. Its growth is a remarkable phenomenon, as is shown in Table III.

TABLE III
HUMAN BRAIN WEIGHT[9]

Newborn	340 gms.
6 months	750 gms.
1 year	970 gms.
2 years	1,150 gms.
3 years	1,200 gms.
6 years	1,250 gms.
9 years	1,300 gms.
12 years	1,350 gms.
20 years	1,400 gms.

It is clear from Table III that while the rate of growth is greatest before birth, the major increase in the size of the human brain occurs soon after birth. The brain nearly triples in size during the first year of life, a growth rate that is not shared by any other animals and that is a direct result of man's placental origin. An infant with a full-sized brain could not be delivered through the female pelvic canal, and yet without a fully developed brain man could probably not have survived as a species. The evolutionary solution to this problem was to delay a major part of brain development until the period immediately following birth. This solution, however, created a new problem. Rapid postnatal growth of the brain requires a sustained supply of appropriate

[9] Calculated from research data obtained by the author at City of Hope National Medical Center, Department of Neurosciences, 1969–71. While this table gives fairly representative values, it must be emphasized that human brain weight varies over wide limits and that size no longer seems to play a major role in evolution. Some very stupid people have very large brains and some brilliant ones have small brains, though a brain of less than 1,000 grams does not seem to be compatible with survival. The brilliant French statesman Léon Gambetta (1838–82) had only a 1,100-gram brain, while Lord Byron's brain weighed more than twice as much (2,350 grams).

nutrients in adequate quantity, without which normal brain development would be jeopardized. No other organism shares this vulnerability with man to the same degree.

But while postnatal growth of the brain is a spectacular event, the prenatal period is even more remarkable. One of the earliest recognizable primordial tissues in the human embryo is the neural plate, the first evidence of cephalization.[10] This is an amazingly early start for brain development, and it may help to explain the brain's extended vulnerability to unfavorable influences, including malnutrition. During the nine months of gestation, the developing brain recapitulates much of the past evolutionary history of the species, all the way from the single cell that emerged some 3 billion years ago, through the various stages of intermediate evolution, to man. This process is as precisely programmed as the building of a complex architectural edifice, with a tyranny of time that cannot be overcome. Each specific part of the structure is scheduled to be completed at a given time and place, and in its proper position in the sequence. The raw materials needed must be available in full and exactly specified measure, and the energy resources must be in readiness to fashion the job. Any failure of logistics is fatal to the brain substructure involved; it will never be properly completed, and the resources will be employed elsewhere and differently, adapting the resulting defect in the least damaging way possible. While a great deal of redundancy, which can mitigate and even overcome a potential defect, is built into the process of growth, a chronic deficiency of resources such as may be caused by malnutrition cannot always be reversed, and a defective substructure will result.

The structures and functions of the brain still defy detailed analysis and complete understanding. Since man first became conscious of his existence, philosophy has been concerned with the nature of the thought processes as well as with the nature of man himself. It has been known since antiquity that the brain was

---

10 A. L. McAlester, op. cit., p. 96.

a unique organ that most likely was the repository of man's divinity and that the frontal lobes behind man's characteristically high forehead were the site of his intellectual superiority. It is that part of the cranial cavity which has expanded the most in hominid evolution, as shown in Figure 1.

Few surgeons or medical investigators dared enter the mysterious confines of the brain, and most of it remained forbidden territory until relatively recent times. This taboo was lifted in the nineteenth century, when the bloody battlefields of Western Europe forced field surgeons to conclude with amazement that men could sometimes survive even with part of the brain shot away.

There is also the story of an American railroad foreman, Phineas Gage, who was immortalized by a strange accident. In September 1848 he was preparing a blasting charge in a rock with a heavy tamping iron when the charge exploded, propelling the 1¼-inch-thick iron rod backward with terrific force. The rod bored completely through Gage's skull from front to rear, and continued beyond for some distance. Gage did not even lose consciousness at the time of the accident. In fact, he was able to walk unassisted and carry on a normal conversation with the physician who attended his wound. Phineas Gage lived for twelve more years and became a legend in medical literature. The remarkable aftereffects of his experience are on the record.* Though there is evidence for some reduction in Gage's mental faculties and particularly for a degradation of his personality, he was able to live a relatively normal life. At autopsy it was found that his brain had suffered severe damage not only in the left frontal lobe, the site of entry of the iron, but also in the right frontal lobe, mainly because of the infection that followed the accident.

These examples dramatically underscore the resiliency, redundancy, and near invulnerability of the mature brain, protected as it is by a rigid bony structure and bathed in a hydraulic medium called the cerebrospinal fluid.

---

* Both Phineas Gage's pierced skull and the heavy tamping iron are on display at Harvard University.

The brain of primates, including man, consists of two lobes, or hemispheres, on each side of the cranium, separated by a deep longitudinal fissure. Though the brain appears as a gel-like, gray-to-pink mass, it is in fact very highly differentiated into many smaller parts, each of which performs specific functions. But, as we have seen in the case of Phineas Gage, at least some of these functions can be transferred to other parts of the brain when normal performance is affected by either damage or destruction.

These many parts divide into two broad segments, the paleocortex (the "old" or primitive brain) and the neocortex (the "new" brain). The proportion of each varies as the evolutionary ladder is climbed. Man's brain is 85 per cent neocortex and only 15 per cent paleocortex. It is in this 15 per cent of the "old" brain that most of the prior history of brain evolution is found. Many of the old functions, such as swimming coordination in the fish and flying coordination in the bird, are still there, buried in the paleocortex. The paleocortex is the control site of the elemental requirements for life: respiration; visceral, spinal, and postural reflexes; movement coordination; regulation and transmission of impulses; hunger, thirst, and sex drives.

But it is the spectacular size of the neocortex that eventually gave man his unique standing on the planet. It is that part of the brain which comprises the frontal lobes and contains the elements of his transcendental advantages in the animal kingdom; it is the site of consciousness, intelligence, and memory.

The mature human brain contains about 11 billion nerve cells (neurons), whose functions are directly related to the acquisition, transfer, processing, analysis, and utilization of information. There are also billions of supporting glial cells, which serve primarily to maintain the integrity of the nerve-cell network and to manufacture an essential fatty structure, myelin.

To generate a human brain of 11 billion neurons requires the production and differentiation of about twenty thousand neurons *per minute* throughout the entire period of prenatal life.[11]

---

[11] C. R. Noback, *The Human Nervous System* (New York: McGraw-Hill Book Co., 1967), p. 65.

These neurons are joined together in a vast entanglement of fibers and filaments that the writer George Gray has called "the great ravelled knot."[12] It is in these woven cellular circuits that the machinery of the brain discharges its unique functions. The brain-neuron complement can be described as a properly interconnected slab 12,000 cells long by 12,000 cells wide by 70 cells thick.[13]

One of the most important properties of the human brain during development is its plasticity, or ability to change and be molded under the influence of the external environment. It is able to receive and use stimuli from the outside during its exceptionally long developmental period. These stimuli can actually cause both structural and functional changes, which will then affect the way the brain will respond to these same stimuli in the future.[14] This is one of the ways in which learning takes place.

While glial cells may be replaced by new cells during the lifetime of the individual, the neurons are not replaced. Humans are born with their full complement of neurons. After birth the brain continues to grow and mature by an increase of glial cells and by addition of the myelin they produce. The neurons migrate to their final location before the maturity of the organism, and with these changes the die is cast. Each and every neuron is as old as the individual; the neurons that die are never replaced. Thus prenatal malnutrition can seriously affect a person's entire life by severely inhibiting the number of neurons produced before birth. This important aspect of the problem will be discussed in a later chapter.

The brain has an extraordinarily high sustained demand for oxygen and nutrients. This is because the brain is never at rest and maintains the same level of utilization of resources whether one is asleep or engaged in highly intellectual activity. Although

12 G. Gray, "The Great Ravelled Knot," *Scientific American*, October 1948.
13 S. Deutsch, *Models of the Nervous System* (New York: John Wiley & Sons, 1967), p. 258.
14 R. J. Harrison and W. Montagna, *Man* (New York: Appleton-Century-Crofts, 1969), p. 95.

the weight of the adult human brain is but 2 per cent of the total body weight, it consumes 20 per cent of the total oxygen (the figure is 50 per cent for the infant) and 20 per cent of the total nutrients of the body. It uses more than 500 calories out of a 2,500-calorie diet, mostly in the form of glucose. To provide this disproportionate amount of body resources, a rich blood supply is carried through the brain; about 800 ml. (1½ pints) of blood flow through the brain every minute. But, paradoxically, the brain has practically no margin of metabolic safety and no reserves. A five-second interruption of blood flow brings unconsciousness, and irreversible damage or death follows a few minutes' deprivation. There exists no good explanation for this puzzling condition. One would logically suppose that this master organ should be able to handle such an emergency. A reasonable answer would seem to be that the extraordinary demands made by the many functions of the human brain are already straining the limits of the relatively small skull cavity. There is neither space nor resource left for anything else, even lifesaving reserves. It is not surprising, therefore, that the complete development of the human brain is essential for the many specialized activities it must continuously carry out. Any impairment of structural or functional integrity will inevitably be accompanied by a substandard level of performance.

Despite this vulnerability to sustained pre- and early postnatal malnutrition, and to oxygen deficiency, the human brain is superbly equipped to resist metabolic assaults from the environment, once it reaches maturity. It has repeatedly been shown that even starvation will cause no permanent damage, and the transitory impairment of functions can be completely reversed once adequate nutrition is re-established.

Thus the biological potential of the human species is derived primarily from the extraordinary competence of the human brain; but this capacity can be approached only when the long, vulnerable, and critical period of development can be allowed to proceed without significant interference.

Chapter III

THE ECOLOGY OF THE WOMB

Throughout the world, four new babies are born every second.

One could assume that medicine devoted to the care of women and children would be the most advanced part of medical research and practice.

Yet nothing could be further from the truth.

The problems of human conception, pregnancy, and birth have received particular attention only in the past half century. Until 1910 there was no organized knowledge in these fields. Gynecology, obstetrics, and pediatrics did not exist as established, separate disciplines of medicine. Only a very few years ago, bright medical students were discouraged from entering these fields and directed instead into such prestigious specialties as surgery.

Throughout history pregnancy and birth were the domain of midwives, whose training was a mixture of practical experience, tradition, and myth. The earliest physicians were more concerned with senility and death than with problems involving the emergence of human life. They were also interested in and puzzled by the epidemic plagues that periodically swept through whole populations only to disappear as suddenly as they had appeared. Often against their wishes, these early physicians were also called upon to repair the human damage brought about by rebellion and war.

These practitioners of the art of medicine (and until recently it was an art with only a small underpinning of science) have been mainly concerned with the ailments that afflict the noted, the noble, and the wealthy, while neglecting the diseases most often found among the poor. It is in this context that the current knowledge of prenatal malnutrition and its effects on brain development must be considered. While it is fairly clear that deficiencies in the ecology of the womb can result in a malnourished fetus,* there remain serious gaps in our understanding of the problem. Taken together, these uncertainties still cloud the conclusions that can be drawn from the scientific evidence.

Contrary to common belief, reflected in the instruction to a pregnant woman to "eat for two," the nutritional and other needs of the fetus are not simply superimposed upon those of the mother. Shortly following conception and migration of the fertilized ovum to the uterus wall, profound changes take place in the body of the mother, by which control of her vital processes is passed to the organism she hosts, the fetus. The ovum, which is by far the largest of all human cells, contains sufficient nutrients to maintain its growth and multiplication for only the first, critical days, during which it moves from its ovary, through the Fallopian tube to the uterus. A week after conception, the developing organism, now floating in the uterus, already consists of several hundred cells, and requires outside nutrients.

At this point, the process of implantation begins, usually on the back wall of the uterus. The colony of cells does not simply attach itself to the uterine wall, but actually digs into it, eroding as it enters, in the manner of an invading parasite. The immediate uterine reaction to this invasion is hostile, but quickly becomes acquiescent; the peace offering comes as a gift of glucose sugar from the mother's stored supply of glycogen. At this point, the

---

* The word "embryo" is applied to the product of conception for the first six weeks of pregnancy, at which time a human resemblance first develops. Thereafter until birth it is generally referred to as the fetus. However, for the sake of simplicity, in these pages the unborn human from conception to birth will be referred to as the fetus.

developing fetus suddenly begins to grow at an explosive rate, in response to the availability of the nutrient. It now doubles in size every twenty-four hours.

This initial supply of glucose, however, rapidly becomes inadequate to support the phenomenal growth rate of the fetus. Something more elaborate is needed to sustain fetal development. This need is met by formation of the chorion (the outer membrane that envelops the fetus), the amnion, and the placenta.

The amnion is a flexible sac filled with a watery medium, the amniotic fluid, in which the fetus floats. This warm and comfortable inland sea is reminiscent of the earth's environment late in the Precambrian era, more than 600 million years ago.

The placenta is a disc-shaped organ in which the blood vessels of the fetus and those of the mother come together in an intertwined mass, without joining. Nutrients, oxygen, hormones, and waste products are exchanged by diffusing from one bloodvessel system to the other. The essential ecological link between the womb and the fetus is the placenta. It is the sole source of nutrients and oxygen from the mother. It manufactures hormones essential for fetal integrity and development, and collects waste products from the fetus to be discharged through the mother's body.

The placenta grows steadily until the seventh month, by which time it reaches full size. When the baby is born, the placenta, delivered as the afterbirth, weighs normally about one pound (500 grams). The vital connection between the fetus and its placenta is the umbilical cord, in which two arteries and one vein carry as much as three hundred quarts of blood per day flowing at the rate of about four miles per hour. It is the placenta which allows the fetus to become an increasingly efficient parasite in its mother's body.

A malnourished mother may be unable to contribute adequately to her placental development. Fetal growth is affected, because a deficient placenta may be unable to keep up with fetal demands for essential nutrients. The best way to determine whether the fetus receives adequate nourishment is to monitor its rate of growth. The classic work of Drs. Robert A. McCance and Elsie M. Widdowson[1] demonstrated that a growing organism is extremely sensitive to variations in nutrition, and that inadequate nutrition, in rats for instance, can have permanent consequences if imposed during critical periods of rapid growth. Their studies showed that early-life undernutrition resulted in permanently smaller animals, even if they later received adequate nutrition for the rest of their lives. Early-life overnutrition produced exactly the opposite effect: permanently larger animals. The same thing is true of human children: children malnourished early in life may be permanently stunted in their growth, even if they later receive a sustained adequate diet.[2] Details of this story will be given in Chapter VII.

Since it is not possible to experiment with pregnant women to determine placental adequacy, animal studies have been the cornerstone of almost all advances in modern medicine and biology. The validity of animal experiments for human beings is based on the simple fact that there are far more similarities than differences between men and animals. There is a great deal in common between an amoeba and a human cell. Much of what is known about human genetics, for instance, has been discovered in studies with garden peas, bread mold, the common fruit fly, and coliform bacteria. Much of the understanding of the biochemistry of human metabolism and respiration has been obtained from bakers' yeast cells, pigeon muscles, and rat livers.

Working with a variety of animals, a number of research teams both in the United States and abroad showed that there exist one or two developmental periods during which there is a rapid "growth spurt" of a particular organ. It is during these times that the availability of nutrients becomes a critical factor. These

---

[1] R. A. McCance and E. M. Widdowson, in *Protein Metabolism*, ed. by F. Gross (Berlin: Springer-Verlag, 1962), p. 109.
[2] M. B. Stoch and P. M. Smithe, "Does Undernutrition During Infancy Inhibit Brain Growth and Subsequent Mental Development?" *Archives of Disease in Childhood* 38 (1963), pp. 546–52.

"growth spurt" periods are predetermined, and they take place according to very rigid schedules of time and sequence. If a scheduled "growth spurt" for a given organ occurs during a period of severe nutritional deficiency, that organ may be permanently stunted for lack of materials needed to develop it. Having missed its scheduled time to develop, it usually never again has the same opportunity to grow. This is why adult malnutrition, with all organs complete and no longer growing, is a fundamentally different problem from child malnutrition. The importance of this difference is only beginning to be appreciated.

A research team headed by Dr. S. Zamenhof, School of Medicine, University of California at Los Angeles, first demonstrated that depriving pregnant rats of protein resulted in a reduced number of brain cells in the offspring.[3] When these animals were fed a diet deficient in proteins (8 per cent instead of a normal 27 per cent), the offspring had a body weight at birth 30 per cent below normal, and a brain-cell count of approximately 10 per cent below normal. In addition, the protein content of these cells was also lower by about 20 per cent. At three months of age the young rats of deprived mothers manifested abnormalities of gait and response to environmental stimuli.

Also working with pregnant rats, Drs. J. K. Stephan and Bacon F. Chow, Johns Hopkins University School of Medicine, and Dr. Myron Winick, Cornell University Medical College, demonstrated that malnourished mothers produced smaller and lighter placentas than adequately fed mothers.[4,5] The difference between these two studies is that the first reported variations in placental weight, while the second showed that there were fewer cells in the malnourished placenta. Both these findings are important, because cell size can change without affecting cell

[3] S. Zamenhof, E. van Marthens, and F. L. Margolis, "DNA (Cell Number) and Protein in Neonatal Brain: Alteration by Maternal Dietary Protein Restriction," *Science* 160 (1968), pp. 322–23.

[4] J. K. Stephan and B. F. Chow, "The Fetus and Placenta in Maternal Dietary Restriction," *Federation Proceedings* 28 (1969), p. 915.

[5] M. Winick, "Cellular Growth in Intrauterine Malnutrition," *Pediatric Clinics of North America* 17 (1970), pp. 69–77.

number. But in both these studies it was evident that the malnourished placenta was not only smaller but also contained fewer cells. *But the most striking finding by Dr. Winick was that newborn animals from deficient placenta also had fewer brain cells.* Therefore, placental inadequacy resulted in inadequate nutrition of the fetus, which affected brain development during its "growth spurt."

It is hard to exaggerate the importance of this observation. It suggests that an inadequate placenta is unable to sustain the availability of sufficient nutrients to the fetus for brain development. Dr. Zamenhof was able to show that an extremely well-developed placenta can work the other way as well. Pregnant rabbits with heavier-than-usual placentas were likely to give birth to animals with a larger-than-normal number of brain cells.[6] Thus the placenta appears to play a crucial role in modulating brain development not only in animals but in humans as well.

Counting billions of brain cells one by one would be an impossible task. An ingenious way of doing this indirectly has been developed. It is based on the fact that each cell of any one species contains the same amount of genetic material (DNA)[†] in its nucleus. DNA is the substance of which all genes in the chromosomes are made; it contains the complete blueprint of the living organism. Each cell of a given species has exactly the same genetic information and therefore contains exactly the same amount and kind of DNA. There exist some exceptional cells, which have a differing amount of DNA, but they are usually too few in number to create problems in the measurement that will now be described. The exact quantity of DNA in each normal cell can be accurately measured in the laboratory. It is also possible to measure the total amount of DNA in a whole organ. Thus by

---

[6] S. Zamenhof, L. Grauel, and E. van Marthens, "Study of Possible Correlations between Prenatal Brain Development and Placental Weight," *Biology of the Neonate* 18 (1971), p. 140.

[†] For a fascinating, human story of the discovery of DNA (deoxyribonucleic acid) read *The Double Helix*, by Nobel laureate and codiscoverer J. D. Watson (New York: Atheneum Publishers, 1968).

dividing the total amount of DNA in that organ by the amount of DNA contained by a single cell, the total number of cells in that organ can be calculated.

This work, together with other research, has generally confirmed that early-life malnutrition in humans and animals results in a decreased number of cells not only in the brain and placenta but in other organs as well. The organs most affected by these nutritional deficiencies are those which have been exposed to malnutrition during the period of their most rapid growth. Even mild malnutrition can result in severe cellular deficits in those organs undergoing their "growth spurt" during that time.

An example of this vulnerability was reported by Dr. J. Dobbing and his collaborators in the Department of Child Health, University of Manchester, England. Pregnant rats exposed to mild undernutrition during the period when the cerebellum portion of the brain was undergoing rapid growth gave birth to animals with a selective and permanent reduction of weight and cell numbers in the cerebellum.[7] The rest of the brain, particularly the cerebral cortex, which grows more slowly during the period of the experiment, showed less pronounced cellular deficit of neurons. Dobbing pointed out in this report that the pattern of cell reduction bore a striking resemblance to that which follows X-ray exposure during this prenatal growth period.

X rays and gamma rays are known to affect cellular replication; this is the principle that underlies cancer radiotherapy. The cells most vulnerable to irradiation are those which multiply rapidly, while those least affected are not. Nutritional deficiency also interferes with cell replication, by reducing the supply of nutrients needed for that process. There is much in common, therefore, between irradiation and nutritional deprivation; the initial cause may be different, but the effect and end result are similar in many respects.

---

[7] J. Dobbing, J. W. Hopewell, and A. Lynch, "Vulnerability of Developing Brain: VII. Permanent Deficit of Neurons in Cerebral and Cerebellar Cortex Following Early Milk Undernutrition," *Experimental Neurology* 32 (1971), pp. 439–47.

Pregnant women are carefully shielded from diagnostic X rays, because such exposure is often sufficient to cause stunted development of the offspring, with the brain the most frequently and most seriously impaired organ. Since brain development starts very early and is terminated very late, irradiation is very likely to stunt development of the brain, which reduces it to a mere useless remnant and results in complete and irremediable mental retardation. This condition is known as microcephalic idiocy.

There are other factors that affect the fetus at different periods or by different mechanisms during pregnancy, and that cause specific damage to organs growing at the time of the insult. German measles (rubella) is usually a mild infection, except during the first trimester of pregnancy. Affected mothers give birth to children with serious eye and ear defects. The apparently innocuous sedative thalidomide (also known by several trade names) was the agent of tragedy in the late 1950s and early 1960s. Women exposed to that drug during the first seven weeks of pregnancy bore offspring who had rudimentary, flipper-like stumps instead of arms and legs but were normal in every other way. It is during the first seven weeks of pregnancy that the "growth spurt" in human limbs takes place.

The human fetal nervous system begins to differentiate very early in pregnancy. On the eighteenth day, the primitive neural plate appears, followed two days later by the rudiments of a forming brain, the visual system, and the central nervous system. By the end of the first month, the head has become the dominant feature the fetus will retain throughout its placental existence. Experiments with rats and other animals have shown that the developing brain is most vulnerable to undernutrition or other insult during the period of maximum growth, and that these restrictions need not be severe to produce permanent deficits. This vulnerable period, while it occurs in both animals and man, varies considerably in the timing of its occurrence. Drs. John Dobbing and Jean Sands studied the development of the human brain by collecting human fetuses resulting from therapeutic abortions, stillbirths, and perinatal deaths and by measuring the DNA content of the whole brain at different periods of pregnancy.[8]

They concluded that there are two major periods of "growth spurt" involving cell multiplication in the human brain; the first occurs between the fifteenth and the twentieth weeks of pregnancy, and the second begins about the twenty-fifth week and continues until the second year after birth. On the basis of considerable prior research, Drs. Dobbing and Sands determined that the first of these two major periods involves primarily neuron multiplication, while the second is predominantly a neuroglial-cell proliferation.

These data provide a new perspective on the nature of the brain defects brought about by fetal malnutrition. This includes incomplete development of one or more parts of the brain, whose stunting depends on the nature, timing, and duration of the malnutrition. It involves not only a decrease in size but also a decrease in the number of neurons, whose multiplication takes place in humans only during pregnancy. This, however, is probably only a limited part of the story.

There are many different kinds of neurons, located in various parts of the brain, and they perform many different functions. The same thing is true of the neuroglia, but not to the same extent, because there are fewer different kinds of neuroglia than of neurons. Evolution has built many safeguards into the organ structure by allowing for fail-safe redundancy. Even though some neurons are known to perform exquisitely specific functions, a large number of them are available to take over those functions in the event of the failure of some of these cells. Phineas Gage's survival is a case in point. But whether this fail-safe mechanism is equally applicable to the developmental stage has not been established with any degree of certainty.

Brain deficiencies resulting from malnutrition may also affect the development of adequate fail-safe redundancy of brain cells by reducing the number of available duplicate cells. Thus a

8 J. Dobbing and J. Sands, "Timing of Neuroblast Multiplication in Developing Human Brain," *Nature* 226 (1970), p. 639.

limited, local failure, which would normally be handled by duplicate cells, cannot be overcome in a brain-cell-deficient individual, and this type of failure, repeated and cumulative, might give rise to mental deficiency. In other instances, when no mental deficiency appears among victims of early-life malnutrition, the stresses that might otherwise exacerbate cellular failure may not have been of sufficient intensity or duration to expose the consequences of cell shortage, and mental performance is not affected. This may explain some of the contradictory results reported by malnutrition-research workers.‡

Protein deprivation is among the most serious forms of early malnutrition, because proteins and the amino acids of which all proteins are made play the most versatile and widespread role in living matter. Drs. Donald F. Caldwell and John A. Churchill, Department of Gynecology and Obstetrics, Wayne State University School of Medicine, Detroit, Michigan, showed in 1967 that the learning ability of rats was significantly decreased when the mother was denied an adequate protein diet during the last part of her pregnancy.[9] Dr. Churchill and his coworkers then investigated this effect in humans by keeping records of poor pregnant black women and their children. In these studies the investigators were very careful to exclude all pregnancies that exhibited evidence of medical or obstetric complications. A professional dietician estimated the amount and kind of food eaten by these women every twenty-four hours. The women were divided into two groups, those whose daily protein intake was greater than 70 grams (2½ oz.) and those whose intake was less than 50 grams (1¾ oz.). Since even under these controlled

‡ A word of caution, however, must be added. This conception of a fail-safe redundancy mechanism is only a speculative possibility that is intended merely to illustrate how reduced numbers of brain cells might affect cognitive faculties. Future research will undoubtedly offer other explanations, but this one at least has the virtue of simplicity and is based on what is already known about brain functions.

[9] D. F. Caldwell and J. A. Churchill, "Learning Ability in the Progeny of Rats Administered a Protein-deficient Diet During the Second Half of Gestation," *Neurology* 17 (1967), p. 95.

conditions it is difficult to be sure that the dietary information given by these women was accurate, blood samples were regularly taken and analyzed for circulating amino acids, the breakdown product of protein ingestion.

The results of this study were an extraordinary confirmation of the influence of diet. The researchers observed a striking relationship between the amount of amino acids in the bloodstream of pregnant women and the birth weight and skull volume of the offspring. Mothers who had less than 4 mg. per cent* of amino acids in their blood bore children who weighed less than and had smaller skulls than those of mothers whose blood had more than 4 mg. per cent amino acids. The duration of pregnancy was about the same for both groups. Premature births therefore played no role in the observed results.[10]

The relationship between low birth weight and mental retardation has been established by numerous investigators as long ago as 1919.[11,12] But the interpretation usually given was that premature birth was an important cause of mental retardation. This kind of explanation, while probably valid in part, obscured the effect of malnutrition on subsequent mental retardation. In fact, some investigators in this field showed that some of the most severely mentally retarded children were the least premature.[13,14]

Dr. Churchill found that retarded children have a low weight

---

* Blood substances are often measured in milligrams per cent. This means the weight of the substance in milligrams found in each 100 milliliters of blood. There are 65 milligrams in one grain U.S. avoirdupois; 100 milliliters is about 3½ fluid ounces.

[10] J. A. Churchill et al., "Relationships of Maternal Amino Acid Blood Levels to Fetal Development," Obstetrics and Gynecology 33 (1969), p. 492.

[11] A. Ylppo, "Zür Physiologie, Klinik und zum Schicksal der Frühgeborenen," Zeitschrift für Kinderheilkunde 24 (1919), p. 1.

[12] A. Capper, "The Fate and Development of the Immature and the Premature Child," American Journal of Diseases of Children 35 (1928), p. 262.

[13] J. Douglas, "Mental Ability and School Achievement of Premature Children at Eight Years of Age," British Medical Journal 1 (1956), p. 1210.

[14] D. Baird, "The Contribution of Obstetrical Factors to Serious Physical and Mental Handicap in Children," Obstetrics and Gynecology of the British Empire 66 (1959), p. 743.

at birth, and that most of those he studied were born at term.[15] Such low-birth-weight children born at term are usually designated as "small-for-date." These findings were confirmed by other investigators.[16] Dr. Churchill, among others, suspected that a significant portion of the mentally retarded population was composed of full-term individuals who until recently would automatically have been described as premature. It is always a tricky business to establish conception date, and the given date of the last menstrual period is notoriously unreliable for calculating the length of the gestation period. It has been commonly assumed by most physicians that an underweight baby at birth is probably premature, when in fact that child may have gone through a full-length gestation but suffered from malnutrition.

Dr. Churchill undertook to make a careful study of this important question by investigating twin births. His reasoning was that twins tax maternal resources much more severely than does a single fetus, and that since one twin often manages to do better than the other during gestation, this fact should be reflected in a significant difference in mental ability. Since both twins are exposed to the same environment for the same length of time, any mental difference between them, if related to birth weight, should be an important observation indeed.

It is known that twins are often small at birth even when carried to term, and there are considerably more mental retardates among twins than among single births.[17,18] It is also known that placental blood circulation is not shared equally by even identical twins.[19]

---

[15] E. Bandera and J. Churchill, "Prematurity and Neurological Disorders," *Henry Ford Hospital Bulletin* 9 (1961), p. 414.
[16] J. Warkany, B. B. Monroe, and B. S. Sutherland, "Intrauterine Growth Retardation," *American Journal of Diseases of Children* 102 (1961), p. 127.
[17] J. Berg and B. Kirman, "The Mentally Defective Twin," *British Medical Journal* 1 (1960), p. 1911.
[18] R. Illingworth and G. Wood, "The Incidence of Twins in Cerebral Palsy and Mental Retardation," *Archives of Diseases in Childhood* 35 (1950), p. 332.
[19] B. Price, "Primary Biases in Twin Studies," *American Journal of Human Genetics* 2 (1950), p. 293.

Dr. Churchill selected fifty pairs of twins among 116 referred to the Psychologic Clinic of the Detroit public school system between 1960 and 1963 because of learning problems. They ranged in age from five to fifteen. Their histories were carefully examined both from the original hospital birth records and from information given by the mother about the pregnancy, birth, and postnatal life. The children were given physical and neurological examinations as well as the intelligence test known as the Wechsler Intelligence Scale for Children (WISC).† In Dr. Churchill's statistical analysis of these fifty pairs of twins, the mean full-scale I.Q. of the heavier twin was 81.9, while that of the lighter one was 78.6. This difference was found to be statistically significant.‡ [20]

This important work has been abundantly confirmed by other investigators. In 1969, for instance, Dr. Linda C. Eaves and her team of Canadian researchers from the departments of Psychiatry and of Pediatrics, University of British Columbia, Vancouver, B.C., reported on the I.Q. test scores of children with a low birth weight.[21] The 502 children selected for this study were all born in the Vancouver General Hospital, and all had a subnormal birth weight: less than 2,000 grams (4½ lb.). These children were compared with 207 normal children, born in the same hospital, whose birth weight was greater than 2,500 grams (5½ lb.), and whose social-class distribution reflected the cross section of the low-birth-weight children.

Both the low-birth-weight and the normal children were given a battery of medical, psychiatric, and I.Q. tests over a period of eighteen months. Some children were dropped from these

---

† This I.Q. test and others are explained in detail in Chapter VI.

‡ The statistical significance of this difference was expressed by saying that the probability factor, p, was less than 0.05. This means that the probability of this difference's being due to pure chance only is less than one in twenty.

[20] J. A. Churchill, "The Relationship Between Intelligence and Birth Weight in Twins," *Neurology* 15 (1965), pp. 341–47.

[21] L. C. Eaves *et al.*, "Developmental and Psychological Test Scores in Children of Low Birth Weight," *Pediatrics* 45 (1970), p. 9.

46   THE MALNOURISHED MIND

studies when it was found that they had either an extremely low
I.Q. (below 50), a major brain defect, deafness, or blindness.

The results of this study showed that children with low birth
weight consistently scored lower than normal children. The truly
premature among them generally scored even lower than the
small-for-date children, but not consistently so. Dr. Eaves's group
also noted that this correlation of I.Q. deficiency with low birth
weight became less distinct as the child's age increased from two
and one half to four years.

But socioeconomic status played an important role in I.Q. deficiency, becoming more significant with increasing age. For low-
birth-weight children, at six months of age there was only a
five-point spread in I.Q. scores between the highest and the lowest socioeconomic classes. At two and one half years of age the
spread had grown to thirteen, and by age four it had reached
seventeen points. But when these low-birth-weight children were
compared with normal children of comparable social background,
the normal children still performed significantly better than did
their weight-deficient counterparts. This last observation is of
capital importance. It suggests that socioeconomic status alone
does not account for differences in the performance of these children and that the prenatal environment must therefore have
played an important, if not a crucial, role. When low socioeconomic status is superimposed on low birth weight, it compounds
the difficulties already experienced by these children.

Another significant study is that of Dr. D. J. P. Barker, Department of Social Medicine, University of Birmingham, England.[22]
His observations were made on a group of 606 mentally subnormal children drawn from a population of 73,687 single births for
which medical records were available. These 606 children were
between nine and fourteen years of age, and their I.Q. on a
standard Stanford-Binet test* was less than 75, while the mean

22 D. J. P. Barker, "Low Intelligence. Its Relation to Length of Gestation
and Rate of Fetal Growth," *British Journal of Preventive Social Medicine*
20 (1966), p. 58.
* This and other I.Q. tests will be discussed in Chapter VI.

value is 100. To eliminate cases of mental deficiency resulting from clear-cut causes such as birth trauma, only those subnormal children for whom there was no known cause were selected for this study.

Dr. Barker divided the 606 children into three groups according to their I.Q. scores (below 50, 50–64, and 65–74), and compared their birth weight and the length of their mother's pregnancy with these scores. The findings from this study are clear; at all levels of intelligence the mean birth weight of the mentally subnormal children was low compared with that of children of normal intelligence. Yet 71 per cent of the children were born in the normal period of between thirty-nine and forty-one weeks of pregnancy. But since their birth weight was lower than normal, the inference was that the rate of growth of these fetuses was slower than normal.

Small-for-date as well as premature children do not reach their full biological potential, either physical or mental, no matter how well they are fed in later years. Such investigators as Dr. Cecil M. Drillien, Department of Child Life and Health, University of Edinburgh, Scotland, have made thorough analyses of small-for-date children. Dr. Drillien has shown that there is among these children a much higher incidence of mental and physical handicaps than among normal children, and that the severity of these handicaps rises rapidly with decreasing birth weight. The numbers are dramatic; while only less than 1 per cent of normal children exhibited mental difficulties, that figure rose to an astounding 54 per cent for children with a birth weight of 1,360 grams (3 lb.) or less.[23]

Until recently it was an accepted fact that dietary deficiencies resulted in the stunting of the body as a whole. Emphasis has now been shifted to the recognition that the brain is particularly vulnerable to damage from early-life malnutrition. This emphasis has been reflected in such reports as that of Drs. Heinz F. Eichenwald and Peggy Cooke Fry, Department of Pediatrics,

[23] C. M. Drillien, *The Growth and Development of the Prematurely Born Infant* (Baltimore: Williams & Wilkins, 1964), p. 215.

University of Texas Southwest Medical School, Dallas.[24] Drs. Eichenwald and Fry point out, "It has long been scientifically acceptable, and in some circles even fashionable, to ascribe many behavioral characteristics of the older child and adult to conditioning experiences received during infancy and perhaps prenatally."

These behavioral characteristics probably have a biochemical rather than an environmental conditioning basis. The best-studied aspect of this "biochemical conditioning" is nutrition and its deficiencies. When adequate nutrition is withheld, physical development is suppressed simultaneously with the biochemical development upon which it depends. This has been shown to occur in both children and experimental animals, and to affect a wide range of processes, including water distribution, fat absorption, and concentration of blood lipids. The retention and excretion of a number of metabolic products sometimes mimics inborn-error-of-metabolism diseases, such as PKU (phenylketonuria), with all their mental-retardation consequences. In reviewing his own work as well as that of his colleagues elsewhere, Dr. Drillien concluded, however, that the most likely effect of retarded intrauterine growth could be a general lowering of intelligence as determined by I.Q. tests, rather than the production of severe handicaps.

Such handicaps, when they arise, may be due to congenital factors rather than to malnutrition, and their inclusion in these studies has obscured the results.[25] Low-birth-weight, premature, and small-for-date children are born in large numbers throughout the world, and not all of them can be ascribed to the nutritional status of the mother. But these infants are more prone to biochemical deficiencies, such as a reduced level of glucose in the blood. A shortage of glucose in the blood of these children trans-

[24] H. F. Eichenwald and P. C. Fry, "Nutrition and Learning. Inadequate Nutrition in Infancy May Result in Permanent Impairment of Mental Function," *Science* 163 (1969), p. 644. Copyright 1969 by the American Association for the Advancement of Science. Quoted by permission.
[25] C. M. Drillien, "The Small-for-Date Infant: Etiology and Prognosis," *Pediatric Clinics of North America* 17 (1970), p. 9.

lates into a glucose shortage for the developing brain, and this is a possible cause of brain damage.[26]

Similarly, the cause-and-effect relationship between prenatal malnutrition and mental retardation may not be immediately obvious. The nature and duration of malnutrition appear to be extremely important in the production of observable brain damage. For example, Dr. Peter Gruenwald and a group of Japanese collaborators[27] studied the mean birth weight of Japanese infants over the twenty-year period between the wretched conditions prevailing in Japan at the time of its surrender at the end of World War II to the years of relative affluence following the remarkable rebirth of that country in the mid-1960s. These investigators found not more than a 10 per cent difference in birth weights during that period.

The frightful famine of the winter of 1944–45 in the Netherlands, during which pregnant women's weight gain was reduced from twelve to only two kilograms, reduced their offsprings' mean birth weight by only some 7 per cent. A group of investigators from New York State Department of Mental Hygiene Epidemiology Research Unit I, Division of Epidemiology, Columbia University School of Public Health and Administrative Medicine, reported that Dutch women pregnant during this wartime famine gave birth to children whose mental performance at age nineteen did not seem to be related to that exposure.[28]

An explanation for these apparent discrepancies, however, may not be so difficult to find. Both Japan and the Netherlands have been affluent nations with excellent nutrition, except for a short, acute period. Pregnant women, therefore, can be presumed to have had ample reserves and to have maintained an adequate

---

[26] S. L. Manocha, *Malnutrition and Retarded Human Development* (Springfield, Ill.: Charles C. Thomas, 1972), p. 186.

[27] P. Gruenwald *et al.*, "Influence of Environmental Factors on Fetal Growth in Man," *Lancet* 1 (1967), p. 1026.

[28] Z. Stein *et al.*, "Nutrition and Mental Performance. Prenatal Exposure to the Dutch Famine of 1944–1945 Seems Not to Be Related to Mental Performance at Age 19," *Science* 178 (1972), p. 708.

fetal nutritional level during the famine. Those women who were not able to maintain this reserve would have been unable to conceive, would have aborted shortly after conception, or would have given birth to a child whose lowered vitality would have brought about an early death.[29]

This has been strikingly demonstrated by Dr. A. N. Antonov, who reported on the children born during the siege of Leningrad in 1942,[30] and by Dr. Clement A. Smith, who reported on children born during the Dutch famine of 1944–45.[31] Dr. Smith points out that what occurred in Holland was a relatively brief period of severe, generalized undernutrition, *not outstandingly poor for any single dietary element*. This he fully documents from the abundant data obtained from the records of the National School of Midwives at Rotterdam and the Obstetrical Service of the Zuidwal Hospital at The Hague, as well as from the Oxford Nutrition Survey carried out under the sponsorship of the Supreme Headquarters, Allied Expeditionary Forces in Europe, and evaluated by Dr. Hugh M. Sinclair.[32]

Mental retardation associated with prenatal malnutrition appears to depend primarily on *chronic* rather than *acute* circumstances. Acute malnutrition of generally well-fed women is not comparable to a history of chronic malnutrition among poor and generally ill-fed mothers.

A number of investigators, notably Dr. Clement A. Smith,[33] have suggested that intrauterine stunting may have a genetic component. This is a difficult hypothesis to verify with any degree

---

[29] C. M. Drillien, "The Small-for-Date Infant: Etiology and Prognosis," *Pediatric Clinics of North America* 17 (1970), p. 9.

[30] A. N. Antonov, "Children Born During the Siege of Leningrad in 1942," trans. from the Russian, *Journal of Pediatrics* 30 (1947), pp. 250–59.

[31] C. A. Smith, "The Effect of Wartime Starvation in Holland upon Pregnancy and Its Products," *American Journal of Obstetrics and Gynecology* 53 (1947), p. 599.

[32] H. M. Sinclair, *Oxford Nutritional Survey*. Preliminary Report on Nutritional Surveys in the Netherlands, May and June 1945 (Oxford).

[33] C. A. Smith, "Prenatal and Neonatal Nutrition," *Pediatrics* 30 (1962), p. 145.

of assurance. But the evidence on identical twins, whose genetic makeup is identical, supports a predominantly environmental hypothesis. Such twins can differ markedly in birth size, and it is the lighter one of the two who is the most likely to exhibit evidence of mental retardation. This difference is observable even many years later. A team headed by Dr. S. Gordon Babson, University of Oregon Medical School and Emanuel Hospital, Portland, Oregon, has followed the growth and development of twins who were dissimilar in size at birth.[34] These investigators made a search for surviving sets of dissimilarly sized twins in the records of two Portland hospitals from 1950 to 1958. They selected those sets of twins whose smaller one was at least 25 per cent smaller and whose weight was less than 2,000 grams (4 lb. 7 oz.) at birth. Sixteen surviving pairs of twins that met the criteria were available for study. They were children between the ages of four years five months and ten years eleven months, with a median age of eight and a half years. Fourteen of the sets were white, one was black, and one was Japanese. The average birth weight of the smaller twin was 1,610 grams (3 lb. ½ oz.), and the larger one averaged 2,470 grams (5 lb. 7 oz.), with an average difference between the twins of one third, or nearly two pounds.

Each set of twins was examined by a pediatrician, a clinical psychologist, a speech pathologist, and a clinical pathologist. To avoid biasing these examiners, information on birth size was withheld from them. The children were also given blood, hearing, speech, and I.Q. tests. The results showed that even eight and a half years, on the average, after birth a significant difference in height, head circumference, weight, and I.Q. was present between the lighter and the heavier twins, with the lighter twin exhibiting a markedly lower-than-normal record. This was true of both fraternal and identical twins.

This study confirmed the early, pioneering work of Dr. Josef Warkany, Children's Hospital Research Foundation, Cincinnati, Ohio. Dr. Warkany and his collaborators studied twenty-two

---

[34] S. G. Babson et al., "Growth and Development of Twins of Dissimilar Size at Birth," Pediatrics 33 (1964), p. 327.

small-for-date children over a long period of time and found only
five of them within the normal I.Q. range.[35]

In addition, Dr. Robert A. McCance, Infantile Malnutrition
Unit, Mulago Hospital, Kampala, Uganda, demonstrated that
the imprint of differential food intake persists even when un-
limited food becomes available at later stages of development.[36]

Thus the evidence indicates the negative effect of prenatal
malnutrition on brain development and on cognitive faculties.
It suggests that part of the damage induced by this nutritional
deficiency is long lasting and may even be permanent. But
whether or not it is permanent is not as important as the fact that
it persists at least long enough to interfere with learning during
the critical, early years and thus interferes with the adaptation
of the child to society. Not only does he bring a deficient mind
to the task of growing up, but he is also condemned to do poorly
in school, with all the consequences this entails for him, his family, and society at large. The longer it takes the child to catch up,
if this is possible at all, the more his chances for a fulfilling life
will have been reduced.

An advance in the field of prenatal malnutrition and its later
consequences comes from the laboratory of Dr. Stephen Zamenhof, Brain Research Institute and Mental Retardation Center,
University of California at Los Angeles.[37] It may have great impact on the argument of nature versus nurture in brain development and cognitive faculties. It will be recalled that Dr.
Zamenhof and his coworkers were able to correlate prenatal brain
development with placental weight. In a continuation of these
studies, female rats were kept on a protein-restricted diet one
month prior to mating, in order to simulate the condition of
chronic malnutrition. These animals were then mated with nor-

35 J. Warkany, B. B. Monroe, and B. S. Sutherland, "Intrauterine Growth
Retardation," American Journal of Diseases of Children 102 (1961), pp.
249–79.
36 R. A. McCance, "Food, growth and time," Lancet 2 (1962), p. 671.
37 S. Zamenhof, E. van Marthens, and L. Grauel, "DNA (Cell Number)
in Neonatal Brain: Second Generation (F_2) Alteration by Maternal (F_0)
Dietary Protein Restriction," Science 172 (1971), p. 850.

mal, well-fed males. After mating, the pregnant females continued to be maintained on the same deficient diet to which they had been exposed earlier. The female offspring of these pregnancies were properly fed either from the time of birth or from weaning to the time of their adulthood, mating, and throughout their pregnancy.

These second-generation rats were studied by Dr. Zamenhof and his team, who observed that even though these second-generation animals were the offspring of well-fed parents, their brains were smaller and the brain-cell number was significantly lower than normal, just as in the case of their malnourished grandparents. The explanation given by Dr. Zamenhof for this striking result is based on the observation that a young malnourished female will later, when pregnant, be unable to develop an adequate placenta. An inadequate placenta will be unable to sustain the level of nutrient the fetus requires for normal growth.

Thus Dr. Zamenhof's group has opened the door to knowledge of an unexpected consequence of malnutrition. Their studies showed that the influence of malnutrition, including mental retardation, may extend beyond the malnourished parents and their offspring to the second generation, even though this second generation is well fed throughout its life.

The significance of their finding is further strengthened by a previous study carried out by Drs. J. J. Cowley and R. D. Griesel, University of Natal, South Africa.[38] In one experiment, rats were fed a low-protein diet. Their offspring were rehabilitated by weaning to a higher-protein diet, and then tested for mental ability. In another experiment, the *second* generation of low-protein-diet rats was fed the rehabilitation diet from weaning, and their offspring were tested for mental ability. Rat performance can be measured by mazes and other tests to determine problem-solving ability. The results of these experiments showed that (1) retardation became more marked as successive generations

---

[38] J. J. Cowley and R. D. Griesel, "The Effect on Growth and Behavior of Rehabilitating First- and Second-Generation Low-Protein Rats," *Animal Behavior* 14 (1966), pp. 506–17.

of rats were reared on the low-protein diet; (2) a low-protein diet fed to one generation of rats affects the growth and development of the next and possibly the subsequent generation as well; (3) in rehabilitating low-protein rats, *more than one generation* may have to be fed an adequate diet before all the effects of the low-protein diet can be overcome.

If it can be confirmed that these observations apply to humans as well as to rats, then a major new consequence of malnutrition will have been uncovered; that is, the damaging effects of prenatal malnutrition can operate *for at least two generations* to simulate the influence of heredity, even though the proximate cause is environmental.

None of the studies relating malnutrition to brain development has as yet taken this possibility into consideration, nor has any of the studies purporting to relate I.Q. to hereditary factors. With continuing research, there is likely to be a downward revision of the view current among some psychologists that as much as 80 per cent of the I.Q. potential is contributed by heredity while the remainder is the result of environmental influence.

Dr. Christopher Jencks and his associates in the Graduate School of Education, Harvard University, have reassessed the effect of family and schooling in America, including the contribution of heredity to I.Q. Dr. Jencks concludes that this factor most probably ranges around 50 per cent,[39] which is already a substantially lower figure than 80 per cent. And even then, Dr. Jencks is careful to point out, the data base on which such calculations are made is still too weak to justify a precise estimate. Indeed, these estimates make no provision at all for such factors as malnutrition and its possible effects across generations, independent of any genetic factor. When it becomes possible to make meaningful estimates of these influences, it is likely that even Dr. Jencks's revised estimates of the genetic component will be found to be on the high side. A further discussion of this point will be found in the last chapter of this book.

---

[39] C. Jencks *et al.*, *Inequality, A Reassessment of the Effect of Family and Schooling in America* (New York: Basic Books, 1972), p. 315.

In a review article, Dr. G. A. Neligan, Department of Child Health, University of Newcastle upon Tyne, Great Britain, has summarized the conclusions of his studies on the effects of intrauterine malnutrition on the later behavior of children as follows: "It must be said at once that the results all point in the same direction, suggesting that there is an adverse effect upon intelligence and emotional development—however difficult it may be in individual studies to eliminate or allow for the effects of associated perinatal factors or those of associated adverse environmental factors in later childhood."[40]

Dr. Neligan's own work confirmed the existence of the tendency of "light for date" babies to show inferior subsequent development. This was reflected in a significantly lower height, weight, and I.Q. among these children when tested at the age of five. The lower the birth weight of the baby, the sharper the deficiencies observed five years later.[41]

Nothing has been written here, and very little can be found in the research literature, about the influence of malnutrition on the father's role in conception. But there is evidence that suggests such an influence exists. Malnutrition may seriously interfere with the production of viable sperm cells in both men and animals.[42] There are also reports that provide evidence for the possibility that not only the nutrition of the mother and the mother's mother may be involved in the development of the fetus, but also that of the mother's father.[43, 44]

The surface of knowledge on this subject has barely been

---

[40] G. A. Neligan, "The Effects of Intrauterine Malnutrition upon Later Development in Humans," *Psychiatria, Neurologia, Neurochirurgia* 74 (1971), p. 453. Quoted by permission.

[41] G. A. Neligan, "The Clinical Effects of Being Light for Date," *Proceedings of the Royal Society of Medicine* 60 (1967), p. 881.

[42] H. Stieve, *Der Einfluss des Nervensystems auf Bau und Tatigkeit der Geschlechtsorgane des Menschen* (Stuttgart: Georg Thieme, 1951).

[43] A. Montagu, *Prenatal Influences* (Springfield, Ill.: Charles C. Thomas, 1962).

[44] H. G. Birch and J. D. Gussow, *Disadvantaged Children* (New York: Grune & Stratton, 1969).

scratched, and the subject has not yet received the attention it deserves, scientific research being a dirty word in both state and federal governmental circles today. But there is little doubt that prenatal malnutrition is strongly associated with the impairment of mental abilities in later childhood.

Yet this is only part of the story. The other part deals with the effects of early-life malnutrition on young children, about which much more is known than about prenatal factors. A prenatally malnourished fetus is bad enough, but a prenatally malnourished fetus followed by a malnourished infant is infinitely worse, and the two almost always go together. In fact, prenatal malnutrition may predispose an infant to particularly severe consequences if he is exposed to postnatal malnutrition as well.[45] We will learn more about this in the following chapters.

---

[45] J. A. Brasel and M. Winick, "Maternal Nutrition and Prenatal Growth," *Archives of Diseases in Childhood* 47 (1972), pp. 479–85.

Chapter IV

HUNGER, MALNUTRITION, AND STARVATION

Fifty miles south of Hamburg, Germany, lie the twin villages of Bergen and Belsen, site of the infamous concentration camp of Bergen-Belsen during World War II. On April 12, 1945, the victorious British Army reached the horror camp and liberated fifty-five thousand still-surviving but starving inmates, many of them near death. A few days later a group of medical experts armed with special food and equipment were flown in to save as many camp victims as possible. Thousands were dying from starvation as hospital accommodations were improvised and patients brought in, many moribund, for special treatment. Predigested proteins were given by intravenous injection, and when this made the patient's condition worse, these nutrients were given instead by mouth, only to be found unpalatable.

The reaction of the patients to these efforts was one of undisguised horror. It seemed to them that their saviors were continuing, with added savagery, the tortures initiated by their Nazi captors. Many died during these well-meaning but clumsy attempts at salvation, but in the process it was discovered that the best treatment was to feed them skimmed milk by mouth. Not one of the experts had foreseen that predigested protein foods might not serve their purpose or that skimmed milk would be the treatment of choice. Fortunately, however, very large supplies of skimmed-milk powder were stocked behind the advancing Canadian lines, and they were made available to the starving populations of western Holland also. Experience with skimmed milk there confirmed the findings made at Bergen-Belsen at such frightful human cost.

This incredible story, reported by one of the distinguished experts on the scene, Sir Jack Drummond, underscores the abysmal ignorance of human nutrition still rampant in the middle of the twentieth century. Said Drummond in conclusion:

"Although in our lifetimes millions have died from starvation . . . it was not possible to find clear-cut advice [on] how to resuscitate people who are near death from this cause. That fact is, I think, a terrible reflection on our lack of concern for the human race as a whole."[1]

This lack of concern continues to be expressed in many ways, beginning with the startling fact that it is still extremely difficult to document the existence of malnutrition in the United States. The report by a distinguished Citizens' Board of Inquiry into malnutrition in the United States, entitled *Hunger, USA*,[2] made a serious indictment of the appalling dearth of information available to the health professions and public officials. Until 1968, for instance, the *total extent* of medical knowledge about dietary intake and malnutrition among the poor was derived from approximately thirty studies. The scope and methodology of these studies, with a few exceptions, left much to be desired. They usually focused on areas convenient to the location of the medical school doing the study, thus bypassing essential data on the nutritional status of specific and critical segments of the population.

Medical schools still do not treat malnutrition as a regular

---

[1] J. Drummond, *Problems of Malnutrition and Starvation During the War*, Sir Jesse Boot Foundation Lecture, University College, Nottingham, England (1946), pp. 17–18.
[2] Citizens' Board of Inquiry into Hunger and Malnutrition in the United States, *Hunger, USA* (Boston: Beacon Press, 1968).

subject for study, investigation, or medical training. Most physicians, in fact, are unable to recognize and diagnose it except in those obvious cases where medical training is not necessary, i.e., gross underweight or overweight. Clinical aspects of nutrition are usually not taught as a separate discipline, and the few courses on the subject that do exist are usually inadequate to the task.

Most hospitals do not keep meaningful records or perform clinical tests to identify malnutrition. The Citizens' Board of Inquiry into Hunger and Malnutrition in the United States reported that it had requested each state board of health to determine how many cases of malnutrition or deficiency disease were diagnosed in its hospitals in a given year. Ten states ignored the request, and thirty-five of the remaining forty replied that they did not keep such records. Many of them explained that they assigned the reason for the hospital stay or the primary cause of death to some other factor, even though this factor may have been brought on by lowered resistance to disease caused by malnutrition.

Most American experts in malnutrition among the poor have acquired their specialty by studying the problem in foreign countries, almost always with a U. S. Government research grant or with a subsidy from a domestic foundation. The nutritional problems of the poor in this country have been almost completely ignored. In the decade 1956–66, for instance, the Interdepartmental Committee on Nutrition for National Development (ICNND), an office of the Public Health Service, was responsible for funding thirty-three studies, thirty-one of which were carried out in underdeveloped nations of the world and only two in the Indian reservations of the United States. The Citizens' Board of Inquiry into Hunger and Malnutrition in the United States reports that it visited the Office of Economic Opportunity library early in its study and found not one word of information on malnutrition in the United States—this in the one agency of the U. S. Government most directly concerned with the problem!

Dr. Jean Mayer, Professor of Nutrition, Harvard University, was one of the first to appear before the U. S. Senate Select Committee on Nutrition and Human Needs in 1968. His testimony is a serious indictment of the medical profession. It includes the following statement:

Let me say to the national policymakers here that I think they have no reason to blame themselves for not knowing what has not been brought to their attention by the professionals who should have done so. Not enough attention has been focused on malnutrition by the medical profession. Important though nutrition is, both in the case of the poor or [sic] in the case of the rich, in terms of prevention of coronary disease, it has been all too often ignored by our doctors.

By and large, nutrition is still not taught or properly taught in the medical schools of this country. Most medical schools have no nutritionists as such.

There is no awareness of the need for a systematic teaching of nutrition. When a professor of obstetrics talks about the care of pregnant women he will say something about nutrition; when a professor of pediatrics will talk about babies, he talks about malnutrition. But there is usually no over-all, coordinated study of the subject.

A department of nutrition, when it exists, is usually in schools of public health, agriculture, [or] home economics, but not in medical schools.

Policymakers are used to hearing about health problems through the medical profession, and the lack of interest of the medical profession in nutrition is certainly one of the major reasons why policymakers have not heard more about the problems of malnutrition.

Now what I am talking about are, for instance, studies on anemia. I take this example because yesterday I was looking at a paper submitted by medical research workers in Detroit on the hemoglobin levels of babies.

I think arbitrarily the distinction between what they call anemic babies and nonanemic babies was put at 10 grams of hemoglobin. Ten grams for babies is not a high level.

The reason they took that distinction is that they were dealing with an entire population which is low in hemoglobin.

This was a paper in a very poor area in Detroit and they just adjusted their criterion of normality so that they would end up with 20 percent of the children characterized as abnormal rather than 80 or 90 percent.

Now this was not a bad paper but it was fairly characteristic of the weaknesses of many of our studies: there was no discussion as to why everybody was so low, what are the factors that led to this. Instead an arbitrary criterion was set up, sort of ad hoc, and a comparison was initiated between babies who were worse off with babies who are better off nutritionally.[3]

Anemias are a complex group of diseases in which the oxygen-carrying, circulating red blood cells are deficient in quality or quantity or both. Anemias are among the many specific conditions that are brought about by malnutrition and that may affect mental capacity and the ability to learn. The red substance of the red blood cells is the protein hemoglobin, in which most of the iron in the body is found. Hemoglobin in the red blood cell is central to the transport of oxygen from the lungs to every part of the body. While the muscles can store oxygen, the brain is unable to do so, as we have seen, and is therefore critically dependent on a sustained oxygen supply.

The muscles store oxygen in another iron-containing protein, myoglobin, and make it available for use during muscular contractions. Each and every living cell has other iron-containing substances, the cytochromes. They are involved in the ultimate chemical process by which oxygen is "burned" to water with the production of biochemical energy for all living processes. Iron, therefore, plays many crucial roles in living organisms.

As the child grows rapidly in his early years of life, his need for iron grows rapidly also. Iron is needed for building new red blood cells as well as for replacing old ones, since the average life expectancy of a red blood cell is only four months. Much of the iron from the old red blood cells is recycled for use in the manufacture of new ones, but the over-all need for additional iron remains very high. Good evidence for this comes from experiments with rats. When rapidly growing fourteen-day-old nursing rats are denied an iron-rich diet through their mother's food supply, they may develop severe anemia within a week. If

[3] *Nutrition and Human Needs,* Hearings before U. S. Senate Select Committee on Nutrition and Human Needs, 90th Cong., 2nd sess., December 1968, Part 1, "Problems and Prospects" (Washington: U. S. Government Printing Office, 1969), p. 27.

this deficiency is continued for three to five weeks past weaning, growth retardation develops.[4]

A number of studies have shown that lack of sufficient iron in the early years of life has a negative effect on mental functions. While the effect of iron deficiency on I.Q. (intelligence quotient as measured by I.Q. tests) is relatively small, the attention span of anemic children was found to be markedly lower than that of normal children. They exhibited more aimless manipulation, less complex and purposeful activity, and were able to perceive fewer stimuli in the presence of other, dominant stimuli.[5]

In short, the anemic children exhibited evidence of symptoms associated with severe impairment of learning ability. It should be emphasized that the serious reduction of attention span in children is almost always associated with poor scores on intelligence tests. And these children are for the most part residents of poor urban and southern rural ghetto areas, in which blacks and Spanish-speaking minorities represent the majority of inhabitants.[6]

Food is a basic element for survival in life. Yet this fact is so distant from American middle-class concern that descriptions of the horrors of food deprivation have little or no emotional impact on most of us. Hunger, malnutrition, and starvation are ideas that require a major effort of the imagination to conjure. In the daily assault of news from distant lands, these concepts are devoid of interest when they are not a total bore. Most of us can hardly imagine ever being touched by them. Some probably even feel an indistinct satisfaction in the fact that some of the inhabitants of this overpopulated planet are thus reduced to silence, an anonymous swarm of unwanted human beings whose sole contribution is to the world's already excessive burden of misery.

Although the words "hunger," "malnutrition," and "starvation"

---

[4] P. R. Dallman, "Significance of Iron Deficiencies," in *Extent and Meanings of Iron Deficiencies in the U.S.* (Washington: Food and Nutrition Board, National Academy of Sciences, 1971), p. 77.
[5] D. Howell, "Consequences of Mild Deficiency in Children," ibid., p. 65.
[6] W. Shubert, "Infants," ibid., p. 9.

are often used interchangeably, they actually mean different things.

Hunger is the group of symptoms that arise from the depletion of food in the body. These symptoms disappear rapidly when the physiological and psychological deficit of nutrients has been made up. We know very little about the very complex processes that go on in the body, and particularly in the brain, either to initiate or to stop the hunger syndrome. We do not know why the hunger pangs stop even before food digestion has made nutrients available to the body. Neither do we know how some animals know instinctively what to eat, and in what proportions, to stay alive and healthy. We do know that human beings are born with some positive instincts in this respect, but that these are quickly extinguished by environment and training. It is believed that one part of the brain, the amygdala, plays a role in the capacity to discriminate among foods. When it is surgically removed from the temporal lobe of the brain of a dog or a monkey, the animal's ability to choose among foods is partially lost, even though removal of the amygdala does not affect the sense of smell. An animal may smell the odor of spoiled food, for example, but its brain will not interpret this odor in a way to cause the animal to avoid eating it.

The best working definition of malnutrition is that used by the U. S. Senate Select Committee on Nutrition and Human Needs: "Malnutrition is an impairment or risk of impairment to mental and physical health resulting from the failure to meet the total nutrient requirements of an individual."[7] This definition is particularly significant because it reflects recognition that the brain can be impaired by malnutrition.

Excessive intake of food leading to obesity, high blood pressure, and related disease normally comes under the heading of malnutrition. However, in this book the word "malnutrition" re-

---

[7] *The Food Gap: Poverty and Malnutrition in the United States,* Interim Report prepared by Select Committee on Nutrition and Human Needs, U. S. Senate, August 1969 (Washington: U. S. Government Printing Office, 1969), p. 8.

fers to nutritional deficiency only. In our prepackaged-food culture many people eat excessively of overprocessed foods and as a consequence suffer from deficiency malnutrition. Physicians see an increasing number of babies suffering because of their teenage mothers' diet of potato chips and cola drinks. Deficiency malnutrition among the affluent but nutritionally illiterate middle class is a major problem, which deserves attention; however, it is a story beyond the scope of this book.

Starvation is the most extreme form of malnutrition. Famine, the starvation of whole populations, has recurred throughout the whole of recorded history. The first reference to famine and its cure can be found at the beginning of the Old Testament, when the thirty-year-old Joseph becomes the Hebrew adviser to the Pharaoh of Egypt:

> And the seven years of dearth began to come, according as Joseph had said: and the dearth was in all lands; but in all the land of Egypt there was bread.
> And when all the land of Egypt was famished, the people cried to Pharaoh for bread: and Pharaoh said unto all the Egyptians, Go unto Joseph; what he saith to you, do. (Genesis 41:54–55)

Much of human history has been involved with the search for and the production, protection, and assurance of an adequate food supply. Advances of civilization have always been associated with the development of agriculture, which increased food productivity so that societies could diversify labor and devote time to pursuits other than those necessary for survival. Progress, therefore, can only be measured by the ease with which the necessities of life can be obtained. Today the achievement of centuries of effort is once again threatened by the huge increase in world population. The number of people starving today is greater than the total population of the earth at the time of the American Revolution. Jules Michelet, the great historian and author of *The History of the Nineteenth Century,* wrote that no one will ever understand that period until a terrible book has been written: *The History of Hunger.*

The many famines recorded in ancient chronicles include the Roman famine of 436 B.C., during which thousands of people committed suicide by throwing themselves into the Tiber River, which flows through the city of Rome. Egypt, which depends on the Nile River and its fertile delta for its agriculture, suffered many such severe episodes, but probably none worse than the great famine of A.D. 42, during which a great part of its population was wiped out.

India, whose rivers also play a crucial role in maintaining its agricultural lands, is heavily dependent on rainfall. During the great Indian famine of 1344-45 the Mogul emperor was unable to provide the barest necessities for his own household. There was no rainfall at all during the terrible years of 1660 and 1661 on the Indian subcontinent. Less than a century later more than 10 million people, a third of the total population of Bengal, are said to have perished during the famine of 1769-70. More than 5 million persons died between 1876 and 1878 in Bombay, Madras, and Mysore, despite frantic but pitifully inadequate attempts to prevent it.[8,9]

Famines were common in Europe as well. Between A.D. 1000 and 1880, one hundred fifty famines occurred in Europe—one every six years.[10] The failure of the potato crop, the main food staple of Ireland, in 1846 and 1847 was caused by a fungus blight. It was responsible for the death of nearly 3 million people and led to the massive Irish emigration to the United States, which played such a major role in subsequent U.S. political history.

William Farr, a mathematician of the nineteenth century, wrote:

In the XIth and XIIth century [in England] famine is recorded every 14 years, on an average, and the people suffered 20 years of famine in

---

[8] C. Walford, *Famines of the World, Past and Present* (New York: Burt Franklin, 1970, reprint of 1879 edition).

[9] Encyclopaedia Britannica, Vol. 9 (Chicago: Encyclopaedia Britannica Press, 1965), p. 58.

[10] R. Dumont and B. Rosier, *The Hungry Future,* translated by R. Linell and R. B. Sutcliffe (New York: Frederick A. Praeger, 1969), p. 23.

200 years. In the XIIIth century the list exhibits the same proportion of famine; the addition of five years of high price makes the proportion greater. Upon the whole, scarcities decreased during the three following centuries; but the average from 1201 to 1600 is the same, namely, seven famines and ten years of famine in a century. This is the law regulating scarcities in England.[11]

While most famines have been caused by crop failure, drought, disease, pestilence, floods, earthquakes, and other natural disasters, many have been induced by inhumanity in war and civil disturbance. None of these, however, approaches for sheer savagery the infamous policies of the German Third Reich between 1933 and 1945. Among the many documents that have survived from this period, few equal in chilling quality the memoranda relating to planned starvation of whole populations, such as the secret one dated May 1, 1941, seven weeks before the German invasion of the U.S.S.R., which states: "There is no doubt that as a result, many millions of persons will be starved to death, if we take out of the country the things necessary for us."[12]

The Nazi governor of the Warsaw district, in Poland, is quoted as having said in 1941, upon the sealing of the nine square miles of that city that were to house half a million Jews: "The Jews will disappear because of hunger and need, and nothing will remain of the Jewish question but a cemetery."[13] Only a few hundred survived after a month of fighting prior to the ghetto's total liquidation, on May 16, 1943. One official order, dated April 19, 1941, was preserved from this period. It reads: "The basic provisioning of the Jewish Residential District [the official euphe-

---

[11] W. Farr, "The Influence of Scarcities and the High Price of Wheat on the Mortality of the People of England," *Journal of the Royal Statistical Society* IX (1846), p. 158.
[12] Nuremberg Trials, Nazi Conspiracy and Aggression, Memorandum of Meeting V, p. 378 (N.D. 2718-PS), quoted in W. L. Shirer, *The Rise and Fall of the Third Reich* (New York: Simon & Schuster, 1960), p. 833.
[13] J. Apenszlak, ed., *The Black Book of Polish Jewry* (New York: American Federation for Polish Jews in Cooperation with Association of Jewish Refugees and Immigrants from Poland, 1943), p. 22.

mism for the Warsaw ghetto] must be less than the minimum necessary for preserving life, regardless of the consequences."[14]

Slavic and Jewish *untermenschen* (subhumans) were exterminated in planned campaigns of starvation by withholding "the things necessary for us." Thus nutritional discrimination became the handmaiden of racial discrimination, and tens of millions of human beings perished in the process.

While there exist numerous early records of famine and its medical consequences, the data are scant and scattered and contain very little useful information. The reports that came out of World War II, however, are somewhat more useful, because an enormous number of people were incarcerated for one reason or another, medical observations were more sophisticated, and in some cases systematic records of inmates were kept.

But even these records, voluminous and detailed as some of them are, do not go beyond qualitative descriptions and are thus very disappointing to the careful investigator. In the few cases in which solid quantitative observations were made, the circumstances under which the data were gathered made it impossible to collect all the information necessary for drawing meaningful conclusions. The siege of Leningrad, between November 1941 and April 1942, yielded numerous biochemical studies, especially during the subsequent period of recovery (spring and summer 1942), but because of fuel shortage, power failures, and constant disruption caused by military action, few meaningful records were kept during the most severe period of the terrible winter of 1941.[15]

Among the studies of starvation that date from the bleak period of Nazi hegemony, none were carried out with greater care or scientific objectivity than those which heroic scientists

[14] "Economic Sector of Jewish Residential District of Warsaw, Order of April 19, 1941 (German document), *Bleter far Geschichte* (Warsaw, Poland: Jewish Historical Institute) XII (1959), p. 65, quoted in L. Tushnet, *The Uses of Adversity* (New York: Thomas Yoseloff, 1966), p. 22.
[15] A. N. Antonov, "Children Born During the Siege of Leningrad in 1942," *Journal of Pediatrics* 30 (1947), pp. 250–59.

and physicians of the Warsaw ghetto carried out in 1941–43 under conditions of wholesale human extermination. Among their observations were instances of brain damage in starving young children.[16]

It is only since World War II that systematic studies on human malnutrition and starvation have been done at the level of scientific objectivity and scope necessary to yield significant conclusions. However, one earlier study, dating back to World War I, deserves mention.

Between 1917 and 1918 an experiment was carried out with human volunteers at the Carnegie Nutrition Laboratory, in Boston.[17] The fatal flaw in this historically important experiment was that the degree of total weight reduction aimed for and achieved in the young volunteers was limited to 10 per cent over a period of several months. The planners of the experiment believed that this amount of loss would be sufficient to learn a great deal about changes in the various functions of the body under food-intake restriction resembling that of a famine. The investigators were also anxious to assure the volunteers that no hazard to health would result, thus essentially vitiating their original purpose and unwittingly defending the concept that a 10 per cent loss of weight was perfectly compatible with the maintenance of good health. Obviously the circumstances of the Carnegie Nutrition Laboratory Experiment were far removed from the conditions of real starvation.

In 1944, under the leadership of Dr. Ancel B. Keys at the University of Minnesota School of Public Health, a major study on the biology of human starvation was undertaken using conscientious objectors to military service as volunteers for the most ambi-

---

[16] L. Tushnet, *The Uses of Adversity* (New York: Thomas Yoseloff, 1966). This little book is a masterpiece of restrained and solidly documented data on the circumstances of the research on starvation carried out in the Warsaw ghetto. It is highly recommended reading.

[17] F. G. Benedict, W. R. Miles, P. Roth, and H. M. Smith, *Human Vitality and Efficiency Under Prolonged Restricted Diet* (Washington: Carnegie Institute, 1919), 701 pp.

tious experiment of its kind ever devised.[18] Rigid criteria were used to select volunteers. They had to be in good physical and mental health, with a good health history. They had to be highly motivated, with a willingness to accept acute and prolonged discomfort and a deep and abiding interest and personal sense of responsibility in bettering the nutritional status of famine victims by contributing to scientific knowledge. The thirty-two young men who were finally chosen were in continuous residence at the Laboratory of Physiological Hygiene from November 19, 1944, through October 20, 1945. Some of these men were kept under medical surveillance and rehabilitation for as long as another year. From November 19, 1944, through February 11, 1945, a period of twelve weeks, the volunteers were kept on a strict control diet consisting of an appetizing and varied 3,492 calories per day with adequate and balanced quantities of proteins, fats, carbohydrates, minerals, and vitamins. They were given batteries of physiological and psychological tests as well as X rays and complete dental care.

On February 12, 1945, the semistarvation period of the experiment began. For the next twenty-four weeks, until July 28, 1945, the diet was drastically cut to 1,570 calories per day. Only two meals per day were served, one at eight-thirty in the morning, the second at five in the afternoon. Food was mainly whole-wheat bread, potatoes, and cereals, with considerable amounts of turnips and cabbage. Only minute amounts of meat and dairy products were provided. To allow for individual variations, the diet was either reduced further or increased somewhat to produce the standard 25 per cent weight loss aimed for in the study. The restricted rehabilitation period lasted twelve weeks and ended on October 20, 1945. It was followed by an eight-week unrestricted rehabilitation diet, which ended on December 20, 1945.

To bolster badly sagging morale and break the monotony of

---

[18] A. Keys, J. Brožek, A. Henschel, O. Mickelsen, and H. L. Taylor, *The Biology of Human Starvation* (Minneapolis: University of Minnesota Press, 1950), Vols. I and II.

both the semistarvation and restricted rehabilitation diet, "relief" meals selected by the subjects, but restricted as to amount so as not to damage the experiment, were served on May 26 and September 9, 1945.

The study reports emphasize the appalling inadequacies of our understanding of human nutrition.

Even though the subjects were intelligent, educated persons with good social adjustment, they began to develop symptoms of psychological disturbance by the end of the first month of semistarvation diet. They became irritable, obsessed by thoughts of food, and deeply concerned about their health. They showed discouragement, followed by periods of depression, because of their greatly reduced ability to sustain both mental and physical effort. Toward the end of the semistarvation period, they exhibited the characteristic mask-like, apathetic appearance of victims of starvation. Recovery from semistarvation required almost a year on a full and well-balanced diet; psychological recovery came faster than physical recovery.

What had been observed under real conditions of starvation, notably following World Wars I and II, was now confirmed by the Minnesota study. The subjects expected prompt and complete recovery from the symptoms of starvation during the rehabilitation period. When this proved very slow in coming, their depression and irritability became worse than during the semistarvation period. Among the most acute of these symptoms was that of feeling like sick old men, without libido or interest in life. They found it very difficult to shed protective attitudes and habits they had acquired during the semistarvation part of the experiment. Only after rehabilitation produced noticeable improvement, late in that period, did the morale of the volunteers rise.

Anecdotal beliefs, when repeated often enough over a long period of time, are eventually accepted as fact. For many years, medical textbooks on cardiology, physiology, and nutrition, written by specialists in their fields, either assumed or stated that the human heart is resistant to undernutrition. The principle that this idea supports is that there is a natural tendency toward self-protection of vital organs. Unfortunately, this teleological view is not supported by the evidence obtained from the Minnesota study, nor by abundantly documented evidence on both animals and humans dating back to 1923.[19]

The Minnesota study shows that as starvation progresses, the heart becomes progressively weaker and shrinks in size. When body weight of the volunteers decreased by 15.7 per cent, the heart volume decreased by an equal amount. At the end of the semistarvation period, the heart volume had decreased by 17.1 per cent.

A similarly incorrect assumption existed with regard to the brain, also thought to be invulnerable to malnutrition. The Minnesota study showed that while very little brain weight loss arises as a result of starvation, the mature brain is not immune to it. The loss of brain weight is substantial enough in itself, approaching 10 per cent in seriously starved adults. But more significant was the observation that there are subtle alterations of composition, including the substitution of water for some tissues, probably in the same way that other tissues become bloated.[20]

The immediate consequences of a semistarvation diet are relatively straightforward. When an adult is limited to such a diet, the first observable effect is a rapid 25 per cent weight loss—in about two weeks. At that point, unless the food supply is reduced to a still lower level, an equilibrium is reached, which allows the victim to continue for several months on the same diet with little if any additional weight loss or increased danger of succumbing.

However, if the diet is reduced to a lower caloric content during this equilibrium period, weight loss resumes a rapid downward course and the death rate skyrockets. While the body is able to make extraordinary adjustments to severely reduced die-

[19] A. Keys, J. Brőzek, A. Henschel, O. Mickelsen, and H. L. Taylor, *The Biology of Human Starvation* (Minneapolis: University of Minnesota Press, 1950), Vol. I, pp. 198 ff.
[20] P. Chortis, "Tuberculosis and Hunger Edema," *American Review of Tuberculosis* 54 (1946), pp. 219–26.

tary intake, that adjustment is limited to a loss approximately equivalent to 25 per cent of a person's normal body weight, provided that no strenuous activity is undertaken. But since starvation means a severely restricted food supply, strenuous efforts, often in desperate competition with others, are almost always required to obtain what little food may be available. Under these conditions no equilibrium is reached and death follows quickly. There exists no clear-cut level below which real starvation can be differentiated from semistarvation. Particularly important is the level of physical effort. Men on fifteen hundred calories per day, constrained to hard labor are rapidly reduced to living skeletons, unable to carry out the simplest physical and mental tasks.

Accompanying starvation are such physiological symptoms as edema (swelling of tissue) and often severe and sustained diarrhea, which is a frequent prelude to death. Unless starvation is extreme and prolonged, a gradual increase in the diet of starved adults will eventually reverse the downward course. The victim will survive, and regain all or nearly all of his mental capacities.

The Minnesota study was concerned solely with adult malnutrition, but its findings have been incorrectly assumed to apply to children as well. The weight of the accumulated evidence, however, demonstrates that this is a misleading assumption. A growing organism is completely different from a mature one in its nutritional requirements. A mature adult will usually recover completely from near starvation, but a young child will not, and his vulnerable, growing brain will be the most severely affected organ. A fetus, infant, or young child requires nutrients not only to survive but also to grow. And the nearly explosive intensity of that growth, particularly the growth of the brain, must be provided for in addition to the adult requirements for mere survival.

Given these facts, one cannot help wondering that mere survival, let alone growth, is possible for a severely malnourished infant. It is possible, but the biological price paid for such survival and growth often leads to unrelenting misery and human degradation. The concept of the dignity of man will have no meaning until the consequences of early-life malnutrition are recognized.

Why is there so much indifference to this subject of hunger, malnutrition, and starvation, when children and pregnant women, who generate instinctive sympathy and concern from almost everyone, are the most severely affected victims? Dr. Josué de Castro, ex-President of the Executive Council of the Food and Agriculture Organization of the United Nations (FAO), suggests an answer. He writes that history has been dominated by man's struggle for food; yet it is a subject that, like sex, has long been considered shameful, indecent, and dirty. He points out that while there are thousands of publications on war, its causes, and its effects, very little has been written on the human destruction visited by malnutrition, whose consequences are greater than those of all wars and epidemics put together.[21]

The concept of adequate nutrition is highly complex. To understand the significance of malnutrition, it is necessary to analyze nutrition. There is much more to this subject than just food. And much more is involved in attempting to solve the problem than simply making food available to the hungry, as the next chapter will relate.

---

[21] Josué de Castro, *Géopolitique de la Faim* (Paris: Les Éditions Ouvrières, 1952), p. 29.

Chapter V

WE ARE WHAT WE EAT

The great French chemist Antoine Laurent Lavoisier founded the science of nutrition. In a letter written in 1790 to his friend Professor Joseph Black of the University of Edinburgh he first revealed the extent of his major discovery linking respiration to digestion:

"The quantity of oxygen gas consumed, or converted to carbon dioxide, rises during digestion to 1800–1900 [French cubic] inches. . . ."[1]

Unfortunately, less than four years later, in 1794, this great man was guillotined during the insane excesses of the French Revolution, thus stopping short in his fifty-first year an unprecedented series of scientific contributions. A friend commented shortly after his execution: "It took only a second to cut off his head. A hundred years will be insufficient to produce another one like it."

Lavoisier's pioneering research was a start toward the de-

---

[1] Letter written by A. L. Lavoisier to Professor Joseph Black, Dept. of Chemistry and Medicine, University of Edinburgh, on November 19, 1790, translated by the author from the French text published in *British Association for the Advancement of Science*, Part 1 (1871), p. 191.

velopment of the science of biochemistry, which underlies nutrition. Through complex processes, food is converted into body constituents for building, for repairs, and as a source of fuel for life. In the simplest terms, an adult human body consists of the following general components:

Water	61%
Proteins	17%
Fats	14%
Minerals	7%
Carbohydrates	1%

These numbers may vary somewhat depending on age and sex.[2] The most significant variation is found in infants. At birth the water content of the body exceeds 80 per cent; it then drops rapidly to approach the adult level of about 61 per cent at six months of age. By contrast, the fat content of an infant is very low, approximately one third that of an adult.

The remains of a completely burned adult human body yield about ten pounds of ashes, nine pounds of which are largely calcium phosphate from bones, while the remaining one pound contains all the other minerals of the body.

Dietary deficiencies of vital minerals are relatively rare, with the exception of iodine and iron. In areas where the drinking water is low in iodine, such as Switzerland and the Great Lakes region of the United States, an endemic disease known as goiter is found. Its obvious symptom is an enlargement of the thyroid gland from a normal weight of about an ounce to as much as two pounds. The thyroid gland manufactures an important hormone, thyroxin, which contains iodine. A chronic deficiency of thyroxin in children results in severe mental retardation.

The human body contains about ten gallons of water—61 per cent of the weight of the average adult. Four gallons are in the blood, lymph, and cerebrospinal fluids. The other six gallons

[2] E. M. Widdowson, R. A. McCance, and C. M. Spray, "The Chemical Composition of the Human Body," *Clinical Science* 10 (1951), p. 113.

are distributed among the 50 million billion (5×10^{16}) cells that make up the average adult human body.*

Carbohydrates are commonly considered to be the major body-energy fuel in the diet. This is not quite correct. The source of immediate energy for the brain is the carbohydrate glucose; but the non-esterified fatty acids (NEFA),† rather than glucose, make up the primary fuel reserve of the body. Dr. Vincent P. Dole of the Rockefeller University in New York has calculated that NEFA can be mobilized to provide body energy two and one half times faster than glucose.[3] Body carbohydrate reserves are found mostly in the liver and muscles in a complex storage form of glucose known as glycogen, which is in fact animal starch. Cellulose, the undigestible roughage of plants, is also a substance made up of glucose molecules, but humans are unable to metabolize it. Cows and other herbivores, however, have stomachs (rumens) full of specialized bacteria that can break down cellulose into glucose.

It is not surprising, then, that carbohydrate reserves in the human body add up to less than 340 grams (¾ lb.).[4] Fats can be mobilized and converted into carbohydrates by some of the most elaborate and exquisitely controlled biochemical reactions known. There are many other sugars besides glucose involved in metabolism, and some of these play important roles. Among them is galactose, a component of the milk sugar lactose, which is a vital factor in the synthesis of myelin, a complex brain fat, during brain development.[5,6]

---

* This number is based on the following assumptions: (1) an average cell weighs 10^{-12} gram; (2) an average adult weighs 60 kilograms, or 132 pounds, and cell weight makes up 81% of the total.

† NEFA are components of fats.

[3] V. P. Dole in *Chemistry of Lipids in Relation to Atherosclerosis*, I. H. Page, ed. (Springfield, Ill.: Charles C. Thomas, 1958), p. 189.

[4] S. Soskin and R. Levine, *Carbohydrate Metabolism*, 2nd ed. (Chicago: University of Chicago Press, 1952).

[5] E. A. Shneour and I. M. Hansen, "Epimerase-catalyzed Glucose-Galactose Interconversion in the Developing Mouse Brain," *Brain Research* 16 (1969), pp. 501–10.

[6] E. A. Shneour, "UDP-Galactose-4-Epimerase Activity of Developing Mouse Brain and Liver Extracts," *Brain Research* 16 (1969), pp. 493–500.

The word "fat" is not a scientifically precise term. A much better word is "lipid." Lipids do not dissolve in water but only in an organic solvent such as wood alcohol, paint thinner, or cleaning fluid. This is a major distinguishing characteristic of lipids, which allows them to perform a myriad of unique functions, many of them related to the protection of the many water-soluble substances that are essential ingredients of living organisms.

Lipids are essential components of membranes. Living cells are complex little bags in which many still smaller bags, called organelles, are found. Organelles perform a variety of specialized biochemical functions without which cells could not exist. Without their separation by membranes, diametrically opposed functions often could not be performed because of mutual interference. The brain is the best example of an organ whose membranes probably contribute to its most complex functions: those of consciousness, thought, and reason. It is mainly during early brain development that most of the more essential membrane structures are formed. Mental retardation may result from the incomplete development of these membranes as a result of nutritional deficiency.

Lipids, therefore, function in at least two essential but distinct ways, first as a major energy store and second as a structural building material. There is still a great deal of controversy over the kind and quantity of lipids that must be included in a good diet, but there is no question that a decent meal cannot be prepared without them. No civilization, whether Eastern or Western, past or present, has been able or willing to forgo them.

During World War II, Great Britain reduced its fat consumption from 39 per cent to 33 per cent, not a very serious restriction. Yet it caused as much public discontent as any of the many other limitations imposed by wartime conditions. After the war, the fat-consumption level rose steadily until it reached the 39 per cent average once again, by the year 1954.[7]

However, even 33 per cent is substantially above the requirement for good health, and desirable life styles cannot be equated

[7] S. Davidson and R. Passmore, *Human Nutrition and Dietetics*, 4th ed. (Baltimore: Williams & Wilkins, 1969), p. 111.

with it. Some societies do relatively well with practically no dietary lipids. A study was made in the early 1940s of the food habits
of an aboriginal people of India, the Hos, in Bihar Province. Two
hundred out of 240 families used no fat at all in the preparation of
food. This was the result of ignorance rather than poverty. The
Hos' cooking was limited to boiling and infrequent baking. They
used cattle solely as beasts of burden and collected from them
neither milk nor meat. Yet they managed well enough so that
none of the symptoms usually associated with fat deficiencies
could be observed. Comparison with other, nearby tribes, who
used vegetable oils in their diet, also failed to reveal meaningful
differences in their health.[8]

This does not mean that the Hos dispensed with all lipids.
There is a small but significant amount of lipids in all foods. With
a few exceptions, all lipids can be manufactured by the human
body; the few that cannot are still essential for life and must therefore be provided from the diet. They are the essential fatty
acids. The human requirements for these fatty acids, however,
are still not established, and it is very hard to find evidence of
a clear-cut role for them.[9] The essential fatty acids are probably
required in extremely small quantities, and most diets probably
provide an adequate supply of them for growth and maintenance.

Lipid dietary requirements provide a striking illustration of
how complex nutritional problems are. This was shown recently
when an attempt was made to alleviate the serious shortage of
protein among South African children. A high-protein diet cured
the protein deficiency but precipitated a serious lipid deficiency.[10] This proved puzzling at first, but careful analysis revealed that since children who suffer from protein deficiency do
not grow, their essential fatty-acid requirement remains very
low. The protein-deficient children therefore appeared to have

---

[8] S. Davidson and R. Passmore, *Human Nutrition and Dietetics*, 4th ed.
(Baltimore: Williams & Wilkins, 1969), p. 112.
[9] *Lipids, Malnutrition and the Developing Brain*, Ciba Foundation Symposium
(Amsterdam and New York: Associated Scientific Publishers, 1972), p. 133.
[10] H. E. Schendel and J. D. Hansen, "Studies on Serum Polyenoic Fatty
Acids in Infants with Kwashiorkor, *South African Medical Journal* 33 (1959),
p. 1005.

a normal complement of essential fatty acids in their bodies, but as soon as sufficient protein became available for them to resume their growth, an increased supply of essential fatty acids became necessary to meet the new demand. Since an adequate supply of these fatty acids was not available in the diet, severe symptoms associated with deficiency of these essential fatty acids soon appeared.

Deficiency of essential fatty acids can cause growth retardation, skin damage, and partial malfunction of many organs, including the brain.[11]

Some of the lipids found in the human body serve as structural material, while the remainder are held as a fuel reserve that can be lost in part without permanent injury. Even some of the proteins contained in the body, perhaps as much as 15 per cent, can be shed by an adult without irreversible damage. A 10 per cent loss of water and a 30 per cent loss of most minerals can also be tolerated. As much as 25 per cent of total body weight can be lost without permanent damage. *But these statements are true only for adults who are no longer growing.* During development and growth of a child, the safety margin is very much smaller, and the consequences of a deficit can be devastating even under mild conditions.

Although proteins make up only 17 per cent of the total body weight and contribute not more than about 15 per cent of the energy requirements, they perform functions whose importance far outweighs their content. Proteins are part of each living cell. They are also key contributors to the structure of cells. Proteins are involved in the many chemical processes that take place within and around cells, including constant repair and replacement. While lipids can be converted to carbohydrates, and carbohydrates can be made from proteins, the reverse is not true; proteins cannot be made from anything except other proteins, and these can arise only from proteins in food.

---

11 *Lipids, Malnutrition and the Developing Brain,* Ciba Foundation Symposium (Amsterdam and New York: Associated Scientific Publishers, 1972), p. 133.

Proteins are composed of some twenty-one different amino acids attached to each other in an almost infinite number of combinations and sizes to yield the most remarkable group of substances in living organisms. They change the rate at which biochemical reactions take place, from days or hours down to fractions of a second. Movement, for instance, would be impossible without fast chemical reactions. As hormones, in extremely minute quantities, they perform amazing biological feats. They can selectively neutralize foreign poisons and can on occasion act as a potent poison themselves, such as snake venom. Antibody proteins can instantly and accurately recognize complex foreign and dangerous antigenic substances and neutralize them selectively. In short, proteins are at the foundation of life itself.

Animals cannot produce the "amino group" (NH_2), the working part of amino acids; these must all eventually be traced back to plants, which can produce the amino group. Plants can make all amino acids from simple inorganic substances in soil, air, and water. Plants are eaten by animals, which in turn make amino acids available to other animals higher on the food chain, up to and including man. While animals cannot make the amino group, they can readily convert one amino acid into another. There are nine exceptions, which human beings cannot manufacture or interchange and which must therefore be obtained from the diet. These are the *essential amino acids,* listed in Table I.

TABLE I

ESSENTIAL AMINO ACIDS FOR HUMANS

1. Histidine (essential only to infants)
2. Isoleucine
3. Leucine
4. Lysine
5. Methionine
6. Phenylalanine
7. Threonine
8. Tryptophan
9. Valine

The amino groups of amino acids contain nitrogen, one of the fundamental elements found in all living things. The essential nitrogen requirement for life can be met with these nine amino acids. They can provide man with all the other amino acids of proteins. Amino acids are building blocks, each with a unique chemical personality. A short description of some of the most interesting among them from the point of view of nutrition, follows:

Glycine: The simplest and smallest, and the most versatile, of all amino acids. During development and growth, the demands for glycine are enormous.

Glutamic acid: The major amino acid of the wheat protein gliadin and an important component of proteins. It contributes a major part of the "meaty" taste of meat. (The meat-taste enhancer monosodium glutamate is simply a salt of glutamic acid.)

Lysine, Threonine: These two essential amino acids figure most prominently in malnutrition, for two reasons: first, they are the most basic of all essential amino acids, because they cannot even exchange their amino group with that of any other amino acid and must be supplied exactly in their original form from the diet; and second, these are the two amino acids in which vegetables, except for peas and beans, are most deficient, and thus the hardest ones to provide from an inexpensive, non-meat diet.

Arginine: Infants may require this amino acid, and it may therefore be an essential amino acid under some circumstances. It is also involved in amino-nitrogen transfers between amino acids.

Cysteine, Cystine, Methionine: These are the three sulfur-containing amino acids. They are found in high concentration in hair and wool proteins. The characteristic smell of burning hair or wool arises from these amino acids. The human body can make cysteine and cystine from methionine, but not the other way around. This places methionine in the ranks of the essential amino acids.

One group of dietary components, the essential amino acids, must be supplied in their original form and cannot be manufactured by the body from other compounds. This fact is most urgently pressing during human development and growth, when the demand for these essential amino acids is immediate and critical.

There is another very important fact about the essential amino acids which is not emphasized in most discussions on the subject, even in scholarly works. This is that the complete group of all eight essential amino acids (or nine in the case of infants) *must be provided simultaneously to the body*. If one is omitted, present in inadequate amount, or administered separately a few hours apart from the rest, the nutritional efficiency of the whole group is drastically impaired. The body, unable to complete protein manufacture, rejects the incomplete set by breaking it down completely and releasing it in the urine in a matter of a few hours. Therefore *the deficiency of a single essential amino acid can be as serious as if the complete set had been omitted from the diet*.

While protein deficiency is perhaps the major nutritional problem facing mankind, there are other dietary inadequacies that have attracted interest and concern and have stimulated the imagination far beyond their actual dietary significance. Vitamin deficiency is the most dramatic and overworked example of this situation.

For many years, especially in the two decades following World War I, the discovery of the vitamins and their almost miraculous ability to cure deficiency diseases dominated scientific and medical thinking. It was argued that nearly all serious nutritional problems could be solved by making vitamins available to everyone. The noted nutritionist Dr. Elmer V. McCollum and his colleagues wrote as late as 1938, ". . . since the necessary experimental procedures are well defined it appears probable that the next one or two decades will witness an essentially complete solution of the present major nutritional problem. This is the discovery of all the essential nutrients for man. . . ."[12]

This love affair with vitamins, abetted by enriched-food processors, vitamin manufacturers and distributors, men of science who ought to know better, infamous writers on nutrition and medicine, and commentators with impressive but phony credentials, has continued unabated to this day. Vitamin pills are need-

---

[12] E. V. McCollum, E. Ovent-Keiles, and H. G. Day, *The Newer Knowledge of Nutrition*, 5th ed. (New York: Macmillan Company, 1938), p. 28.

lessly consumed in enormous quantity by those who often can least afford them. Vitamins are essential in small quantity, and the normal requirement for them is readily available in most diets. Any excess cannot be used and is discarded by the body. In some cases the accumulation of vitamins, particularly vitamins A and D, in tissues can be nefarious.

But vitamin deficiency remains a problem in severely and chronically undernourished children. While its alleviation often produces spectacular results, the importance of vitamins for good nutrition cannot compare with that of the proteins. Nevertheless the discovery of vitamins represents a shining chapter in the annals of biochemistry, which emphasized as nothing else could have done the importance of nutrition in growth and survival. Without going through a descriptive list of all the vitamins, the fascinating stories of some of them will pinpoint the scope of the difficulties faced by the scientists who discovered them, and provide an insight into how dietary problems are solved.

Perhaps the oldest recorded vitamin deficiency involves the dreaded symptoms of scurvy, common among ancient mariners and also the scourge of armies. The symptoms of scurvy usually begin with mental depression and a gradual loss of strength, especially when physical effort is required. This is followed by pallor, sunken eyes, and painful gums and muscles. As the symptoms get worse, teeth fall out and hemorrhages break out in muscles and other tissues, often leaving large visible blotches under the skin. Eventually organs fail and death ensues. But almost up to the point of death, treatment with vitamin-C-containing foods will cause a miraculous and often complete recovery. Many fresh vegetables (particularly cabbages, onions, and carrots) and fresh fruits (especially citrus, such as limes and lemons) are extraordinarily effective in this respect.

English naval history, like that of other nations, is replete with examples of bureaucratic ineptness and stupidity. An example is its treatment of scurvy. The round-the-world mission of 1740–44 under the leadership of Commodore (later Admiral) George

A. Anson was both a military and a medical disaster, from which only the flagship, the *Centurion*, came back to England. Out of 1,955 men who began the journey, only 904 returned, the lost 1,051 having for the most part died of scurvy.[13] This disaster led the Scottish physician James Lind to write a treatise on scurvy, in 1753, in which he pointed out, not without sarcasm, that the antiscorbutic properties of citrus fruits had been known for at least two hundred years before his time. This book was dedicated to Admiral Anson, who in turn appointed Lind to the new Haslar Naval Hospital. Even so, regulations for the use of limes as a scurvy preventative in the British Navy were not promulgated until 1795. The British Board of Trade dragged its feet for another seventy years, until 1865, before introducing a regular ration of citrus juice to the merchant marine, which resulted in the complete elimination of scurvy among its personnel.

This, however, did not prevent Captain Scott of the British Royal Navy from planning an expedition to the South Pole in 1912 without making a single provision for citrus fruits on board. The tragic record of that expedition is mute testimony to the incredible slowness of men to accept even clearly established remedies for their own benefit.

Efforts to isolate the active antiscorbutic factor from citrus fruits were unsuccessful for many years. The first isolation of the pure substance came from the far-removed and apparently unrelated field of biochemistry. This phenomenon is a frequent occurrence in scientific research, a fact that politicians and bureaucrats charged with funding government research are yet to appreciate and effectively exploit. The Hungarian biochemist Albert Szent-Györgyi was working on oxidation reactions in living tissues, in 1928, when he isolated ascorbic acid from animal and plant sources. He proved that this substance was vitamin C, the antiscorbutic factor of citrus fruits, for which he was awarded a Nobel prize in 1937.

In 1912 the English biochemist Frederick J. Hopkins was feed-

---

[13] H. B. T. Somerville, *Commodore Anson's Voyage into the South Seas and Around the World* (London and Toronto: William Heinemann, 1934).

ing young rats a diet of milk protein (casein), lard, sugar, and salts. These animals failed to grow, and died quickly, on that diet. But when Hopkins added only about a half teaspoonful of milk a day, the rats grew well and exhibited vigorous good health. This small amount of milk contributed very few extra calories, which could not possibly have made the difference. Clearly, Hopkins concluded, there was in milk an "accessory factor" that was essential for life and growth. A year later Osborne, Mendel, and McCollum, and independently, Davis, identified the "accessory factor" as a fat-soluble substance they called vitamin A. It is found only in animals, though plants possess substances that can be converted by animals to vitamin A. Liver, egg yolks, dairy products, and leafy or yellow vegetables are all good sources of the potential vitamin. A deficiency of vitamin A in the young inhibits growth and results in damage to the retina and cornea of the eye, eventually leading to complete blindness.

Another interesting story involves the discovery of vitamin B_1, thiamine, one of the so-called B-complex vitamins. While working in a Javanese military hospital in 1890, during the period when the island of Java was under Dutch dominion, the Dutch physician Christian Eijkman was subjected to a typical case of bureaucratic pettiness. Local poultry was being raised on polished rice at the hospital as food for patients suffering from beriberi. Eijkman noted that on this diet the fowls had trouble standing up and could not keep their necks extended. A new chief cook appointed to the military hospital forbade the use for mere fowls of the polished, or luxury, rice ration meant strictly for military use. Instead he fed crude, whole-grain, "civilian" rice to the fowls, which subsequently and miraculously recovered. Eijkman demonstrated that there was something in the outer coating of rice grains that protected chickens from a disease resembling beriberi. For his contribution to the elucidation of beriberi, one of the most intractable diseases of the Orient, Eijkman was eventually awarded a Nobel prize in 1929, sharing it with Sir Frederick J. Hopkins.

Some of the vitamins essential for man are synthesized by

microorganisms that normally live in his large intestine. With inadequate diet, or under other abnormal conditions, these vitamins cannot be produced. For example, a completely vegetarian diet will interfere with the bacterial synthesis of vitamin B_{12} in such a way that neurological symptoms associated with vitamin B_{12} deficiency will often develop. Undernutrition will affect the intestinal flora in the same way, often causing deficiencies of microorganism-produced vitamins. Tapeworms and infections have similar effects, the tapeworm by extracting the vitamins from the food eaten by the victims, and infections not only by affecting the intestinal flora but also by interfering with the absorption of vital components from the digested food.

There is more to food than just nutrition, and only an explanation of this fact will convey the enormous extent of the problem of deficiency as it may affect brain development. What human beings choose to eat is determined not only by the physiological needs of their bodies but also by a formidable array of taboos, superstitions, and conditioning that even rational and technologically sophisticated people accept without question. This problem goes far beyond the problems that scientific research alone can resolve. As in the case of the acceptance of citrus fruit as an antiscorbutic agent, the psychology and the sociology of the problem lag far behind the science. The battle is not only concerned with saving men's bodies; it should be waged to salvage their minds as well.

Food and drink have always had magical implications. Men everywhere are united by food they eat in common. By sharing food with others, we bathe all members of the gathering in an aura of benevolence and peace. In some primitive societies it is believed that casting spells on the remains of food eaten by an enemy can do him serious harm. In our society an undernourished wife will often sacrifice her ration of meat to her husband to keep him strong. Western men will eat raw oysters in the mistaken belief that this will improve their sexual powers.

We assume that the dietary habits of "civilized" nations are rational, while those of primitive tribes are based on superstition. We rationalize our taboos by giving them an aura of logic, when in fact there is none. A good example of this is the belief that Moses' injunction against the eating of pork by the Jews is based on the susceptibility of pork to trichinosis. Thus, runs the myth, this injunction represented an inspired means of maintaining the health of Israel. Recent evidence seriously undermines this comfortable explanation. Abundant quantities of pig bones have been found in prehistoric sites of the Middle East and North Africa, suggesting that pork was eaten in great quantities by the inhabitants of these regions from the earliest times. Pigs were probably the most important domesticated animals of the Sumerians.[14]

So far as trichinosis is concerned, the argument is even more doubtful. The observation of trichinae in muscle requires a high-powered optical microscope for identification, and the pathological symptoms of trichinosis are otherwise so varied that no diagnosis of it is possible without this advanced tool. The most probable reason for the proscription of pork is that the Israelites were nomads, and the raising of pigs is impractical for nomadic people. Pigs are slow and clumsy and cannot be herded over great distances without serious losses.

The Navajo Indians of the United States consider gophers a delicacy, but the chronically meat-deficient poor of the southern states, where gophers abound, would rather starve than consider gopher meat as food. The U. S. Food and Drug Administration has established strong strictures and heavy penalties against the presence of insects in food for human consumption, even though it is impossible to eliminate them entirely. A recent news dispatch from a city in Michigan describes a suit brought by a customer against a supermarket on the grounds that its groceries were infested with cockroaches. The defense won after the supermarket's attorney ate a cockroach in open court with no ill effects.[15]

---

[14] M. Hilyheimer, *Studies in Ancient Oriental Civilizations* (Chicago: University of Chicago Press, 1941), p. 20.

[15] Ann Arbor *News,* Associated Press dispatch, June 27, 1953.

The irrationality of human eating habits is best shown in the history of the edible tubers of the common white, or Irish, potato of Europe and North America. The potato probably originated in the foothills of the Andes, in South America. European visitors to the region in the sixteenth century first thought the potato was a truffle, the rare mushroom used in gastronomic delights. Soon afterward it was used as food on board Spanish ships and brought to Europe. The immediate response to this strange plant was one of deep suspicion. First of all, it was not grown from seeds but from tubers, and no edible plant of that period came from anything but seeds. Secondly, its bulbous appearance was reminiscent of the dreaded lesions of leprosy.

From antiquity through the Middle Ages there evolved a strange but powerful concept of all living things which still exists in some form to this day. This involves the belief that the appearance of a plant or animal provides a clue, or signature, to its medical properties. This superstition was formalized in the early-sixteenth century as the Doctrine of Signatures by a mystic, Theophrastus von Hohenheim (1493–1541), who called himself Paracelsus. The doctrine was further codified by Giambattista della Porta in a book entitled *Phytognomonica,* which was published in Naples in 1588. It focused primarily on the Doctrine of Signatures as it applied to plants.[16] Porta asserted that man could extend his life by eating long-lived plants and shorten it by consuming short-lived ones. This is not so different from "health food stores" today, which sell at very high premium so-called "organically grown" fruits and vegetables, which are green plants. There is no such thing as organically grown plants. All that green plants require to grow on is a supply of water, nitrates, a few minerals, and carbon dioxide from the air through photosynthesis. All these are strictly *inorganic* substances. It is this process of converting inorganic substances to organic ones that makes food available to animals, including man.

It was the Doctrine of Signatures, therefore, that was immedi-

---

[16] A. Arber, *Herbals,* 2nd ed. (Cambridge, England: Cambridge University Press, 1953.

ately applied to the potato; its leprous appearance meant that it should be condemned as a cause of leprosy. Thus, strong opposition to it developed throughout Europe. But as leprosy was then on the wane, that argument gradually weakened and was replaced by a new objection to the potato on the grounds that it was responsible for scrofula, a catchall designation for a wide variety of diseases including tuberculosis, typhoid fever, and typhus. During several of the recurring famines of Europe, many starvation deaths could have been avoided if the potato had not acquired this undeserved infamous reputation.

Among those who set out to combat the prejudices against the potato was Frederick the Great. In 1774 he arranged for a wagonload of potatoes to be sent to the city of Kolberg, Poland, to relieve a developing famine. The response of the citizens was anything but gratitude. They refused to accept the carload of potatoes, sending back a message saying, ". . . those things have neither smell nor taste, and not even dogs will eat them, so what use are they to us?"[17] The Emperor finally broke this opposition by sending a Swabian gendarme to Kolberg who, by eating potatoes in full view of the citizens, convinced them that potatoes were edible and an excellent staple food.

The same problem arose in France, but there the government took a somewhat different tack, more in keeping with the reputation of the French as an eminently logical people. The French Government appealed to the faculty of the School of Medicine in Paris to carry out an investigation of the potato and render a judgment on its merit as food. The faculty dutifully scrutinized the problem and confirmed that the potato was a fine, healthy food with no evidence of any nefarious qualities.[18] Thus did the potato, the undeserved victim of the Doctrine of Signatures, finally gain acceptance in Europe.

---

[17] W. H. Bruford, *Germany in the Eighteenth Century* (Cambridge, England: Cambridge University Press, 1935), p. 116.
[18] R. N. Salaman, *The History and Social Influence of the Potato* (Cambridge, England: Cambridge University Press, 1949), p. 115.

In 1940 a group of American scientists headed by Dr. John Cassel, Department of Epidemiology, School of Public Health, University of North Carolina, studied a Zulu tribe in a native reserve of South Africa. The group's mission was to reduce the huge infant-mortality rate of 276 per 1,000 during the first year of life. Pellagra, a niacin vitamin-deficiency disease, and kwashiorkor, the protein-deficiency disease, were rampant in the population. The scientists made an analysis of the circumstances leading to these conditions and found that maize was the principal staple of the diet. It was prepared in many different and ingenious ways but was rarely accompanied by any other food. The usual drink of the tribe was fermented millet, or millet beer, which was consumed in large quantities all year round. When money was available the women indulged in the purchase of sugar and white bread as special delicacies.

When Dr. Cassel and his colleagues tried to explain to the Zulus that their huge infant-mortality rate was caused by deficient diet, they met strong opposition to change. The Zulu women insisted that this same diet had kept them and their ancestors a strong and virile people. There was not a chance in the world to modify the situation by scientific arguments, and it looked as though modern science had been defeated by a powerful tradition.

But Dr. Cassel was an unusual scientist. He had the wisdom to understand that modern science sometimes has to give way to tradition, and in this case to the history of the Zulu people themselves. He carefully searched the tribal records and found that maize was not an ancestral food at all, but in fact had been introduced by white settlers. Before the advent of the white people, millet, not maize, had been the staple food of the Zulus. They had also been a pastoral people, with large herds of cattle, and had therefore been milk drinkers and meat eaters. They even partook frequently of wild game, fresh fruits, and green vegetables. This was why the Zulus had been a virile and powerful people. Dr. Cassel and his colleagues obtained confirmation of these facts from the elders of the tribe who remembered them, and thus the credibility of the Western scientists was slowly established in the eyes of the Zulus.

But it was one thing for the scientists to gain respect and quite another for them to convince Zulu mothers to drink milk because of its important nutrients. Long-established Zulu taboos prevented pregnant or menstruating women from contact with cattle, because of their supposed evil influence. Superstition held that drinking milk from a cow of another family was equally evil. If a married woman had come from a foreign family, she could safely drink milk only if her father had given her a cow as a wedding present, or if her husband had performed the cleansing ritual of slaughtering a goat. For poor people the opportunity of doing either of these things was non-existent. Dr. Cassel resolved this dilemma by providing powdered milk from a source completely alien to the Zulus. Thus the taboos were broken, and eventually Zulu women accepted fresh milk from the family cows. Twelve years later, the infant-mortality rate had dropped from 276 to 96 per 1,000.[19]

Modern scientific methods are not always advantageous to a primitive people. In 1946 an extensive report was published by a joint team from the Rockefeller Foundation and the Mexican Government School of Hygiene, headed by Dr. Richmond K. Anderson, on the nutritional status and food habits of the Otomi Indians in the Mezquital Valley of Mexico.[20] The Mezquital Valley lies 60 to 120 miles north of Mexico City astride the Pan-American Highway. The altitude of this arid, high plateau region is about 6,500 feet (2,000 meters) and good crops are hard to obtain. Maize and beans are staple foods. Pulque, the potent fermented drink made from the juice of the century plant, is important to both the economy and the nutrition of the Otomis.

In 1941 the Otomi Indians who populated the valley still clung

[19] J. Cassel, "Social and Cultural Implications of Food and Food Habits," *American Journal of Public Health* 47 (1957), pp. 732–40.
[20] R. K. Anderson *et al.*, "A Study of the Nutritional Status and Food Habits of Otomi Indians in the Mezquital Valley of Mexico," *American Journal of Public Health* 36 (1946), pp. 883–903.

to native customs in spite of the influence of the Spanish con-
quistadores of the early-sixteenth century. Though many understood Spanish, most continued to use primarily the Otomi
language. Most of the Otomis lived in small, one-room dirt-
floored huts that leaked badly when it rained. Clothing was
meager, rarely washed, and passed on from parents to children.
Louse infestation was universal because of poverty and scarcity
of water, which had to be brought up with great effort from a
few deep wells. Sanitary facilities and medical care were practically non-existent.

Economically and culturally, the Mezquital Valley was the most
depressed region of Mexico. Yet the Otomi Indians made excellent use of the meager food resources available to them. Every
edible plant was used as food, including many cacti. The Otomi
also consumed a variety of worms and insects, which they ate
with relish. By these means they maintained a diet of considerable variety and nutritional value. Some of the "weeds" the
Otomi used as food proved on analysis to be nutritious and excellent sources of minerals, vitamins, and proteins. Children were
breast-fed, sometimes for several years, and the investigators reported that it was not unusual for a woman to have several children nursing at the same time. Since water was unsafe and hard
to obtain, pulque was drunk in huge quantities by almost everyone, including babies and small children. Some of the men
claimed that it served as a substitute for meat and that they were
unable to work without it.

Because of the extreme aridity of the region, malaria was
almost unknown in the Mezquital Valley. Considering the fact
that the Otomi Indians practiced no dental hygiene, their teeth
were remarkably good; nearly 50 per cent of adult males had
perfect teeth. Pronounced clinical nutritional deficiency was un-
common. Blood studies revealed values that compared favorably
with those encountered elsewhere. The investigators ended their
extraordinary report with the conclusion that the Otomi Indians
had through many centuries developed a way of life and food
habits that were well adapted to the hostile and barren land they

occupied, and that it would be a mistake to attempt to change these habits until their economic and social conditions could be improved.

Preconceived plans to help people nutritionally must be accompanied by a profound and sympathetic understanding of the circumstances involved. Unfortunately, scientists are not always as understanding as Drs. Cassel and Anderson, and, even worse, the government bureaucracies that administer the programs planned by scientists often substitute large sums of money for imagination and sensitivity. The Otomi Indians provide a sobering example of the limitations of our understanding of how nutrition can serve the cause of progress. Often the solution may lie in making full use of locally available resources by patient removal of taboos against certain foods rather than in introducing new and perhaps unsuitable staples from a distant land.

Modern agribusiness and the requirement for economic mass production of foods has drastically diminished the range of edibles that once gave wide variety to meals. Many of the unusual and exotic varieties of food I enjoyed as a child in France are unavailable today even in my native land.

While customs and taboos play a major role in man's relationship to his diet, religion is even more influential. Religion is a powerful, driving force that controls men, and that force is often strong enough to overcome the misery of hunger. Biochemistry and nutrition are therefore not the only significant parts of man's arsenal in the pursuit of a better life, and unless this fact is genuinely understood by responsible leaders, no significant improvement in human nutrition will be possible. We look askance at the Hindu's basic religious belief in which respect for the sanctity of life extends to his cows, even in the face of certain starvation and death. However, in this country and other advanced agricultural nations the government *pays* farmers to refrain from growing or producing foods, while millions of children in these same countries are being doomed by malnutrition to a bleak existence.

In this age of plenty, when modern technology has made it possible to produce food with matchless efficiency, there are proportionally more people who live on the brink of starvation than at any other time in history. There are also more "nutritionists" who render uninformed but influential judgment on food needs and human behavior. There are many documented examples of a little learning's having resulted in needless tragedy and death.[21]

In the 1930s many people became involved in a violent pseudo-scientific controversy in which it was claimed that milk, being a "natural" food, should not be pasteurized, since any interference with its natural state is harmful. Milk is universally recognized as an excellent human food, but it is also an admirable food for microorganisms; it is, in fact, used by bacteriologists as a culture medium for bacteria. As an excellent growth food for bacteria, it can easily become a dangerous vehicle for infections. Unless the greatest care is taken in the handling of milk, it can be readily infected from the cow's udder, from the receptable in which it is collected, from handlers' breathing, sneezing, or coughing into it, or from air-borne pathogens. After standing a short time, it can become a zoo of pathogenic organisms, capable of causing serious disease including tuberculosis, diphtheria, and undulant fever as well as the more common food poisoning caused by salmonellae and staphylococci.

No one in his right mind would be willing to expose any other person, particularly a child, to such formidable risks, especially when these dangerous bacteria can be swiftly and easily destroyed by pasteurization, which involves only fifteen seconds of heating at 72° C (160° F). Yet medical records show that during the period of the battle over pasteurization many children became infected with tuberculosis as a result of the mindless obsession for raw milk. It is even more remarkable to note that this madness is still with us today as a result of the pronouncements of a few misguided but influential speakers and writers on nutrition. In this instance a little learning has indeed been proved to be a dangerous thing.

---

[21] M. Pyke, *Food and Society* (London: John Murray, 1968). This is a remarkable book on mankind's relationship to what he eats. Several of the examples cited in this chapter have been taken from it.

Dr. Graham S. Wilson's book on the pasteurization of milk lists all the arguments advanced by the opponents of pasteurization, people who have nothing to gain from their stand and who bear no ill will to anyone. These even include the claim that the celebrated Pasteur Institute in Paris does not recommend pasteurization, a complete falsehood. All arguments against milk pasteurization are refuted in this book on the basis of strong evidence or upon no contrary evidence.[22] Yet the dispute still goes on unabated. On scientific grounds it is impossible to justify opposition to pasteurization. But it is emotion rather than reason which is involved in this conflict. And human emotion must be recognized as a powerful force that will continue to guide man's actions, particularly in areas which involve him most intimately, such as the food he eats. Therefore nutrition must be concerned with the circumstances under which food is eaten, as well as with what is eaten and in what quantity.

There are no easy solutions to this problem. Solutions must nevertheless be sought, as they were in the case of Cassel's Zulus and Anderson's Otomi Indians, if we are ever to make significant progress in the eventual abolition of the scourge of malnutrition and starvation.

---

[22] G. S. Wilson, *The Pasteurization of Milk* (London: Edward Arnold, 1942).

Chapter VI

THE MEASUREMENT OF
INTELLIGENCE

> "Unfortunate creature! Since my labors
> are wasted and your efforts fruitless, go
> back to your forest and to the taste for
> your primitive existence; or if your wants
> make you dependent on an alien society, go,
> suffer for your misfortune, die of wretchedness
> and boredom at Bicêtre!"*
>
> Jean Marc Gaspard Itard (1775–1838)

Four hundred miles southwest of Paris lies one of the wildest and most rugged regions of France. Consisting of prairies and spectacular mesas and canyons etched by the Lot, Tarn, and Aveyron rivers and softened by tight little forests, this strange and starkly beautiful region has changed little since Roman times. In September 1799, fourteen months after the taking of the Bastille, which signaled the start of the French Revolution, three sportsmen seized a wild, completely naked twelve-year-old boy as he was climbing a tree to escape his pursuers. After a year of handling by various people, he was finally consigned to the care of a young physician, Dr. Jean Marc Gaspard Itard, who headed a deaf-mute institute in Paris.

---

* Bicêtre was an infamous insane asylum in Paris at that time.

This wild boy could produce only inarticulate sounds, ran on all fours, drank water by sucking it like a horse, and possessed what appeared to be a deficient mentality. Itard spent five painstaking and heartbreaking years trying to civilize the Wild Boy of Aveyron. In a moment of frustration Itard spoke the bitter words that begin this chapter. The boy fully understood his mentor; his chest heaved noisily, he shut his eyes and expressed his bitter grief in a stream of tears.[1] While Itard did not succeed in fully rehabilitating the Wild Boy and considered that his long efforts were a failure, he achieved an astonishing amelioration of his condition.

The story of the Wild Boy of Aveyron is not unique. The literature is replete with records of similar cases, of which that of the Wolf-Children of Midnapore (India) is among the best documented.[2] The importance of the Wild Boy of Aveyron is that his story contributed to an awakening of interest in the meaning of mental differences and the recognition that something could be done to help mentally deficient children. Until then it was thought that there was no hope at all of improving their condition.

Today the pendulum has swung to the other side; many specialists believe that with proper supportive training, normal mentation can often be fully restored. The truth probably lies somewhere between these two extremes. Subnormal mental functions resulting from environmental restrictions can probably be overcome in part. But one stumbling block to rational argument about changes in mental capacity lies with the inadequacies of such terms as "intelligence" and "I.Q."

---

[1] Itard's account of his experiences is recorded in two pamphlets, *De l'Éducation d'un Homme Sauvage* (1801) and the more definitive *Rapport sur le Sauvage de l'Aveyron* (1807). Material from these two documents was combined and published as *Rapports et Mémoires sur le Sauvage de L'Aveyron* (Paris: 1894), of which an excellent translation, by George and Muriel Humphrey, *The Wild Boy of Aveyron* (New York: Appleton-Century-Crofts, 1962), exists in the English language.

[2] J. A. L. Singh and R. M. Zingg, *Wolf-Children and Feral Man* (Hamden, Conn.: Archon Books, 1966).

Most people quickly form definite opinions about the mental capacity of their associates. They readily accept the fact that human beings are terribly unequal in this sense. Children, especially, readily brand playmates as "stupid" or "smart." But if they are asked how the determination of intellectual status was arrived at, they offer only vague answers. Adults do not do much better: they assert someone is "behaving like a three-year-old," or to use the favorite exclamation of harassed parents, "Why don't you act your age?" The trouble with this question is that most people do not really know how a three-year-old child is supposed to behave.

To what extent is intelligence affected by environment as opposed to heredity? They both play a role, but it is impossible at present to determine where one ends and the other begins.

A revolutionary advance in our thinking about mental development was made early in this century, by the Swiss psychologist Jean Piaget. For many years Piaget made a systematic observation of children, including his own, and demonstrated the existence of discrete stages in intellectual development.[3] Even though some children reach the various stages earlier or later than others, the sequence of the stages is the same for all children.

The first stage is the *sensory-motor period*. It begins at birth and is usually over before the age of two. During this crucial period the child develops reflexes such as sucking, opening and closing his fists, and kicking his feet. His acts have no goal at first, but gradually become purposeful and involve active exploration of his surroundings. He also becomes conscious that objects exist independently of his awareness. This is one of the reasons why a young child finds so much hilarity in playing peek-a-boo, because he is still not quite sure that what is hidden really exists. By age two, however, he has acquired confidence that it does.

The second stage of development, the *preoperational period,*

[3] J. Piaget, *Six Psychological Studies,* trans. A. Tenzer and D. Elkind (New York: Random House, 1967).

follows the sensory-motor period and usually lasts until age seven. The most important event of this period is the development of the ability to speak and to use language, which involves the use of symbols. This use of language, important as it is, does not confer the ability to manipulate symbols. The child cannot yet reason. Piaget's famous conservation experiment demonstrates this. Two tall, thin glasses are filled with equal amounts of water, and the child agrees that each glass holds the same amount of water. But now, in front of the child, Piaget empties one of the glasses into another, which is short and squat. The child will now insist that the amount of water in the tall, thin glass is not the same as that in the short, squat one. During this period, the world revolves around him; he is completely self-centered and no viewpoint other than his own exists. He thinks that if he closes his eyes during a hide-and-seck game, for instance, he will not be seen.

The next stage is that of *concrete operations*, during which the child begins to think in abstract terms and to manipulate symbols: he begins to reason, to classify people, objects, and concepts into rational structures that Piaget calls groupings. He is quickly aware that pouring a given amount of water from one glass to another of a different shape does not change the quantity of water being transferred, something he could not recognize in the previous period. Piaget calls this an operation: the logical process involved in mentally comparing, transforming, adding, subtracting, multiplying, dividing, and otherwise setting up relationships between things and events.

In the final stage of development, the period of *formal operations* (ages eleven to fifteen), the child not only reorganizes and formalizes abstractions about things and events to include the world around him, but now extends these abstractions into the world of pure reason. The child can imagine water being poured from one glass to another of a different shape without ever having seen the experiment performed. And he will laugh when he is told that younger children think that water changes volume by this process. He can tell the difference between what is real and what is possible. He is also able to invent things and events and manipulate them to yield new relationships—to create. This is, of course, the quality that dramatically differentiates man from other animals.

The importance of Piaget's contribution is that he was able to demonstrate convincingly, through ingenious experiments such as the one involving water transfer, that a child's mental development proceeds through definite and sequential stages suggesting specific biological processes in brain development, the nature of which is still obscure. Piaget's signal contribution has been to show that the child's world and use of intelligence are vastly different from that of the adult, and that this difference must be taken into account in studies involving children.

Perhaps the most essential function of a living thing is its ability to sustain itself and develop by making use of the elements available from the environment. Of these elements, nutrition is the most fundamental. The living organism must adapt to the nutritional environment by transforming what is available into what is required, and the nutrient eventually loses its identity to that of its host. Dr. John Flavell points out that this is a two-way process and that biological adaptation involves an accommodation of an object to an organism as well as the simultaneous accommodation of the organism to the object, and suggests that intelligence, like digestion, is an organized affair with the same kind of interaction with the environment.[4]

There are differences among children in the rate at which they reach Piaget's stages. This indicates that inadequate nutrition

[4] J. H. Flavell, *The Developmental Psychology of Jean Piaget* (Princeton: D. Van Nostrand, 1963), p. 45. Piaget is brilliant as an experimental psychologist but far from lucid in his published work, with the result that the importance of his contribution has not been as broadly appreciated as it should have been. Dr. John Flavell, Professor of Psychology at the University of Rochester, started this book in 1955 with the intention of writing only one chapter of it about Piaget. Flavell's plan evolved slowly before the enormity of the task, and after eight years of work he finally published a 472-page book solely about the psychology of Piaget. It represents a major contribution to the understanding of Piaget's work.

might be associated with regression to an earlier stage, fixation at an intermediate stage, or retardation of advancement to a higher stage.[5,6]

These early developments are related to what we call intelligence. The use of the word itself is of recent origin. The English psychologist Sir Cyril Burt pointed out that this concept, introduced by Sir Francis Galton and Herbert Spencer in the nineteenth century, was not commonly used, and he recalls that he never heard it during his own childhood.[7] As Dr. Harold J. Butcher has pointed out, "intelligence" is a noun, and nouns usually refer to things. Intelligence is clearly not a thing, but rather a sophisticated abstraction for the way people behave. It is much less misleading to think of the concept as the adjective "intelligent" or even as the adverb "intelligently." Once this is understood, however, it is more convenient to use the noun than the adjective or adverb in clumsy circumlocutions. Intelligence, then, is the common characteristic of organisms behaving intelligently.[8] But solving this grammatical problem in the concept of intelligence does not bring us any closer to a definition of intelligence.

Intelligence has been defined in many different ways, and the scientific literature is flooded with contradictory statements about it, which emphasizes how few uncontrovertible facts exist in this field. It should eventually be possible to obtain a meaningful operational definition of intelligence, but in the meantime psychologists have approached it by a process of successive approximations.

Scientific knowledge advances not so much by the directed discovery of new relationships as by gradual and systematic

---

[5] Ibid., p. 417.

[6] M. Laurendeau and A. Pinard, *Causal Thinking in the Child, A Genetic and Experimental Approach* (New York: International Universities Press, 1962), pp. 245 ff. and 276 ff.

[7] C. Burt, "The Meaning and Assessment of Intelligence," *Eugenics Review* 47, No. 2 (1955–56), pp. 81–91.

[8] H. J. Butcher, *Human Intelligence, Its Nature and Assessment* (London: Methuen & Co., 1968), p. 22.

elimination of most of the many possible alternatives. When these alternatives have been reduced to a small number, the correct one often becomes evident in a flash of insight. This is why the history of science is replete with examples of simultaneous discoveries made by scientists unknown to one another and working in laboratories separated by great distances.

It will probably never be possible to define intelligence in a rigorous way, for at least two reasons. The first is the evolving nature of intelligence. It is made up of a very large number of separate abilities, each of which may be independent of the others. Each of us has a different combination of these abilities, each present to a different degree. How does one compare the intelligence of an individual having outstanding verbal skills but poor space perception with that of another individual who cannot express himself well but can design beautiful buildings?

The second is that things difficult to define are even more difficult to measure. An apparently simple measurement, such as the length of an object, can present major technical problems. Objects expand when they are warm and contract when they are cold. The same thing is true for the measuring device, and unless it is made of exactly the same material as the object being measured, the amount of expansion and contraction will be different for each, so that for accurate work the temperature at which the measurement is made must also be precisely chosen.

But in that case temperature must be defined. One must make sure that the object and the measuring device have uniform temperature. Then the unit of length has to be defined. The inch? The centimeter? Quantitation is at the root of scientific research. Unless the matter under study can be measured and the observations described in meaningful numbers, there can be no significant way of making comparisons, expressing relationships, or drawing important conclusions. Therefore the search for assigning precise numbers to observations occupies a major part of the research process. It has already proved very difficult to make what appear to be simple accurate measurements of length. What do we measure when we deal with intelligence, an enormously more complex and considerably more diffuse quantity? A quantity of *what?*

The problem of measuring mental capacity has concerned men for centuries. The first systematic attempt to measure it was made by Sir Francis Galton of England. In 1882 he opened a small laboratory in South Kensington which he named the Anthropometric Laboratory. There he offered, for a nominal fee of threepence, to measure a number of simple physiological responses such as color, vision, hearing acuity, and reaction time, characteristics Galton believed to be associated with what we now call intelligence. Galton opened his laboratory thirteen years after the publication of his famous *Hereditary Genius*, in which he indicated that he was firmly convinced of the natural inequality of men.[9]

Meanwhile James Cattell in the United States was pioneering a more sophisticated series of mental tests, which included memory tests in addition to the measurements devised by Galton. These were primitive tests of simple human responses, which could be correlated with only a few of the factors that make up intelligence.

It is to a French psychologist of genius, Alfred Binet (1857–1911), that we owe the conception and experimentally sound beginning of mental testing. Like Jean Piaget, Alfred Binet was initially trained not as a psychologist but as a biologist. Also like Piaget, he made the observations of his own children the basis of his psychological work. Binet was trained in law and medicine as well as biology. He was not only a great psychologist, a true experimental scientist who based his conclusions on well-conceived and well-performed experiments, but a great humanitarian as well. It was Binet's humanitarianism that gave him a deep concern for the education of mentally retarded children and caused him to be influential in establishing special-instruction classes for them. Until then, no provisions had existed

---

[9] F. Galton, *Hereditary Genius*, An Inquiry into Its Laws and Consequences (London: Macmillan & Co., 1869), p. 339.

for their education, and the rigid French state system of education condemned those who could not measure up to it to the permanent status of wretched outcasts.

Binet was greatly impressed and influenced by Galton's efforts to put mental testing on a sound scientific basis. In 1896 Binet and Victor Henri published an important scientific paper in which they proposed to estimate the mental capacity of school children by the measurement of eleven *facultés* (specific mental abilities). These involved memory, imagination, concentration, comprehension, and appreciation of beauty, as well as conception of ethics and muscular effort, all these presumably controlled by mental processes. This was the beginning of a long and fruitful investigation during which various mental attributes were tested with school children and the results compared with the average school child's scholastic performance at various grade levels. During the following ten years Binet and his colleagues collected an enormous amount of data. With this information Binet was able to determine which of the tests gave a meaningful measure of a school child's ability *as compared with that of other children of the same age.*

Binet's major contribution was providing the means by which a number could be assigned to attributes of intelligence, so that a graded scale could then be devised to estimate the intelligence of school children. For example, Binet found that the ability to remember and repeat a long sequence of numbers forward or backward shows a striking correlation with age, and thus serves as a very effective measurement of "mental age" as compared with "chronological age."

In 1904, mostly at Binet's instigation, the Minister of Public Instruction, an official of great power in the French Government, appointed a commission to determine how to educate retarded children, with Binet as one of its advisers. The commission recommended that special schools be established for these children and that admission to them be decided by mental testing. By 1905 Binet, together with his colleague Théodore Simon, had devised the first formal scale for the identification of mentally retarded children. The testing did not involve assessment of precisely defined *facultés* but represented, rather, an over-all measurement of attributes by a short and simple group testing method. These were revolutionary departures from the past, in which all peripheral criteria (i.e., motor skills, ethics, hearing acuity) were discarded and the ability to exercise good judgment emphasized.

Binet was a brilliant experimental scientist, and an eminently practical man. Spelling out the limitations of his 1905 test scale, he wrote, "Our sole aim is to evaluate the intelligence of retarded children by comparing it to that of normal children of the same age. The study and analysis of their aptitudes we shall reserve for future work."[10] This unshakable intellectual integrity gave him the credibility and moral authority essential to carry on his pioneering efforts with unusual success.

In his experience with mental testing, Binet became aware of many pitfalls of measurement that reduce the potential validity of test results. One of the most important of these involves cross-cultural factors. Another is known by psychologists as the "halo effect," the result of the human tendency to generalize. A preconceived belief in the inferiority or superiority of a person or group, which will affect an examiner in the administration of an intelligence test, is an example of the halo effect. In the testing of groups of dullards, as determined from their school performance, Binet instructed the school authorities to include bright children in the group in order to avoid prejudgment by those administering the test.

The simplicity and attractive numerical expression of the test, as well as its relative success, very quickly caused enthusiasm for it to overshadow the severe limitations that all responsible psychologists from Binet on had warned against. Dr. Lewis M. Terman, for example, noted that even small deviations by an ex-

---

[10] A. Binet and Th. Simon, "Application des Méthodes Nouvelles au Diagnostic du Niveau Intellectuel chez les Enfants Normaux et Anormaux d'Hospice d'École Primaire," *L'Année Psychologique* 11 (1905), pp. 245–66.

aminer from the rigorously defined standard test procedures could produce serious errors in the test results.[11]

I recall a particularly distressing personal experience, in September 1944, when I entered the U. S. Army at Fort Dix, New Jersey. It had been raining in deluge proportions without surcease for days, and the raw recruits were drenched. We were shunted from one watery barracks to another for "processing"— the conversion of a civilian into a military recruit, complete with haircut, uniform, serial number, medical examination, and intelligence tests. Under these numbing conditions, with a sarcastic and decidedly impatient military proctor, I took my intelligence tests. The I.Q. score from these tests is supposed to be a closely guarded secret, but as the large punched-edge cards followed the recruits from one processing station to another there was ample opportunity to peek at those cards. My score was abysmally low. I later had the occasion to take other such tests under more favorable circumstances, and my I.Q. score jumped to a level more in keeping with my self-esteem. The circumstances under which these tests were administered played a major role in the results.

While these intelligence tests, both past and present, have been subject to numerous restrictions in the interpretation of their results, they have been remarkably successful in *predicting* future scholastic or job performance. And it matters not at all whether the test results reflect heredity or environment or both, in whatever proportion; the *predictive ability* of intelligence tests is a demonstrated fact. Therein lies their appeal and popularity. This was, of course, the essential motivation for Binet to develop his test and continue to improve its predictive ability.

The 1905 scale was superseded by greatly improved ones in 1908 and 1911. By then the concept of mental testing was well established, and the original use of Binet's 1905 scale for identification of mentally deficient children for admission to special French schools had been proved an unqualified success.

The Binet-Simon test has undergone many changes and improvements, the most significant of which was its 1916 revision

---

[11] L. M. Terman, *The Measurement of Intelligence* (Boston: Houghton Mifflin, 1916).

by Dr. Terman of Stanford University. The Stanford-Binet test, as this revision came to be known, became the standard intelligence test in the United States.

The term "I.Q." (Intelligence Quotient) expresses in a single number the relationship between the child's actual (chronological) age and his mental age as determined by the test. The intelligence quotient is obtained by dividing the mental age by the chronological age and multiplying the results by 100 to avoid a number with a decimal point. A child of 10 with a mental age of 10 will have an I.Q. of 100. A child of 10 with a mental age of 8 will have an I.Q. of 80, and a child of 10 with a mental age of 12 will have an I.Q. of 120.

Shortly after the publication of the Stanford-Binet test, the United States entered World War I, and the opportunity for the first mass testing arose. The famous U. S. Army Alpha and Beta tests were devised to classify recruits. While these tests served well the purposes for which they were intended, they further solidified after the war the unwarranted belief that mental testing was an unassailable and fully reliable, valid measure of intelligence. In the words of Dr. Florence Goodenough, "The decade of the 1920's was the heyday of the testing movement, the age of innocence when an I.Q. was an I.Q. and few ventured to doubt its omnipotence."[12]

Even though a test score is useful in determining capacity to perform a task involving intelligence, it is not synonymous with that capacity. An I.Q. score does not define intelligence, even though psychologists will on occasion define intelligence as what is measured by an intelligence test. This is, at best, a crude attempt at providing an operational definition for intelligence, and it is, at worst, circular reasoning. When we say that John has an I.Q. of 100 we mean that (1) we have administered an intelligence test to John; (2) we have noted his performance on that particular test; and (3) we have translated this performance into numbers according to clearly defined rules and regulations and converted them by calculation to an I.Q. value of 100. By

---

[12] F. L. Goodenough, *Mental Testing, Its History, Principles and Applications* (New York: Rinehart & Company, 1949), p. 68. Quoted by permission.

comparison with scores on tests given to many children under many diverse circumstances we can, by proper statistical analysis and I.Q. values, draw some conclusions about John's intelligence. But the two are not the same. *Some* elements of what we call intelligence are assessed in I.Q. tests, but there are many more factors encompassed by the word "intelligence" than what is measured by an I.Q. test.

Yet most psychologists when asked will maintain that the I.Q. score does not change with age under normal circumstances. Terman, when introducing his Stanford-Binet revision of the test in 1916, reported very little change in I.Q. scores obtained over a period ranging from days to seven years and used the expression "constancy of the I.Q." But he pointed out later that while half of the children tested showed a change of less than five points, the other half showed much greater change, in a few cases more than twenty points. The I.Q. is *not* constant; it *does change.* However, it is hard to say whether these changes reflect a true change in mental performance, or whether the environmental bias has changed, or both. It is possible, for instance, to coach children in the taking of such tests and thereby improve their test results for a period of as long as three years.[13]

There are many studies on the issue of the constancy of I.Q., of which perhaps the best series was carried out over several years by Dr. K. P. Bradway. She tested children under the age of six, and retested them ten years later. Her results showed that 25 per cent of the children had an I.Q. change of as much as fifteen points, causing her to warn that intelligence tests of young children must be interpreted with great caution.[14] Her results

---

[13] K. B. Greene, "The Influence of Specialized Training on Tests of General Intelligence," in *The Twenty-Seventh Yearbook of the National Society for the Study of Education* (Bloomington, Ill.: Public School Publishing Co., 1928), Chapter 21.

[14] K. P. Bradway, "I.Q. Constancy on the Revised Stanford-Binet from the Pre-school to the Junior High School Level," *Journal of Genetic Psychology* 65 (1944), pp. 197–217. Also see Bradway, "An Experimental Study of Factors Associated with Stanford-Binet I.Q. Changes from the Pre-school to the Junior High School," ibid. 66 (1945), pp. 107–28.

approximated those of Piaget on the change in mental development of children. Both investigators raise many questions about the validity of I.Q. tests as a measure of mental ability, either native or acquired.

Most I.Q. tests are conceptually derived from the Stanford-Binet, and several of the more recent ones have attempted to overcome its weaknesses. An example of a serious Stanford-Binet weakness is the following. Using this test, the I.Q. is calculated by dividing mental age by chronological age and converting that number to a percentage figure. Using this type of calculation, as the chronological age increases the I.Q. will steadily drop. A person with an I.Q. score of 100 at age twenty would drop to 50 at age forty, assuming no increase in mental age and no change in intelligent behavior. This is an unwelcome if not an absurd conclusion.

To overcome this problem, as well as others, particularly in the adaptation of I.Q. testing for adults, Dr. David Wechsler of the Bellevue Medical Center in New York developed a new series of tests beginning in 1939, leading to the Wechsler Intelligence Scale for Children (WISC) in 1949 and the Wechsler Adult Intelligence Scale (WAIS) in 1955.[15] These have since been in use throughout the world.

This test consists of a battery of sub-tests, each of which samples a different criterion of intelligence. This includes explaining the meaning of words, arranging picture cards in a logical sequence to tell a coherent story, determining from a list which things are alike, and doing mental arithmetic.

Scoring the Wechsler tests is different from scoring the Binet tests. Instead of relating mental age to chronological age, the results of the Wechsler tests are compared with those obtained from an appropriate reference population. The average score of the reference population is set at 100, and any deviation from the average is scored above or below that value. This then becomes the I.Q. score.

---

[15] D. Wechsler, *The Measurement of Adult Intelligence* (Baltimore: Williams & Wilkins, rev. 1944).

These Wechsler tests, like all other I.Q. tests, have been criticized on numerous grounds. Dr. William M. Littell emphasizes that the tests have no adequate rationale, that they are yet to be placed on a firm theoretical foundation, and that the lack of investigation of their predictive validity is "appalling." Littell further comments that factors other than those related to intelligence affect the results. He concludes, however, that they merit further research and development.[16]

A major problem is selecting appropriate reference populations to obtain a normal score, especially of black and other minority-group children. This has been especially serious for children in the southern part of the United States. Littell quotes studies involving children who are not retarded by any acceptable criteria or in the judgment of knowledgeable observers, and yet whose average I.Q. is below 70 on the "normal" WISC scale.[17]

The Wechsler method of scoring for I.Q. makes use of the terms "percentile" and "percentile rank." These can be explained as follows. Take a population (large group) of people who have taken an intelligence test. Divide them, according to their performance, into 100 groups. Line up these groups with the lowest-scoring one (1) on the left, and the highest-scoring one (100) on the right. When this is done, you will observe that the groups at each end of the line are extremely small and that those in the middle are the largest of all. If you now draw a chalk mark anywhere on that line, say at group number 40, you will have placed a boundary that will separate all the worst from all the best performers along that line and for that population. The 40th percentile is the point at which 40 per cent of the population has done worse than and 60 per cent has done better than those at the chalk-mark boundary. Similarly, the percentile rank scored by a given child indicates the percentage of those who do no better than he. If a child has a percentile rank of 20, it means that

---

[16] W. M. Littell, "The Wechsler Intelligence Scale for Children, A Review of a Decade of Research," *Psychology Bulletin* 57 (1960), pp. 132–62.
[17] Ibid.

20 per cent of all children tested do not do better than he, but that 80 per cent of them do. I.Q. is different from percentile rank. An I.Q. of 100 is equal to a percentile rank of 50; 50 per cent do better and 50 per cent do no better.

The fact that statistical sampling is involved means that the results can be only as good as the methods used to do the sampling. Political polls have presented a dramatic example of this point. Unless the pollsters carefully select those whom they ask about their political preference, and repeat the polling frequently, they often end up making embarrassing mistakes. Although there have been great improvements in sampling techniques, a very involved and complicated technical art, the results exhibit serious errors. The notorious Literary Digest poll of 1936, which predicted an overwhelming victory for Alf Landon over Franklin Roosevelt on the basis of more than two million straw ballots, and the sophisticated Gallup poll of 1948 projecting Thomas Dewey as the winner over Harry Truman are two of many cases in which gross errors in sampling led to erroneous results. And yet political polls have made use of sophisticated technology, and some of the intelligence tests have yet to emulate them.

Gurkha is a small town in Nepal whose name has been loosely applied to all Nepalese soldiers serving with the British Indian Army, regardless of caste and language. They are an intelligent and martial group, whose prowess is internationally known. The British Army used special mental tests to select the recruits, and Dr. Francis W. Warburton graphically describes the Gurkha recruits' response to this procedure. They exhibited a singular lack of pep, with slow and deliberate movements. "They just plodded solemnly along." They listened to instruction attentively, but with poker faces. There was no sulking or frustration at difficult questions. There was ample co-operation, with amiable demeanor throughout.

While the British troops taking these examinations were competitive and responded with dispatch, the Gurkhas, confronted with what they thought was a speed test, jumbled everything in

a meaningless way but managed to finish in record time. In everything else they did, they were extremely slow and deliberate. Yet
the Gurkhas were doing their best, and their morale was high.
Warburton concludes that people brought up in an environment
less competitive than ours do not reflect their true mental ability
under test conditions. They are not accustomed to concentrating
on such tasks and are not strongly motivated to succeed in
them.[18] The way the Gurkhas approached the situation when
confronted with an abstract test is not unique to them. Assessment of their potential for specific military duty required the
development of tests specially designed for them, and this was
done.

Testing blacks and other groups with different social mores
and experience poses the same kind of dilemma. Psychologists
have unsuccessfully attempted to devise a universal test suitable
for all human beings. Their attempt has failed because social and
ethnic factors cannot be fully eliminated. It thus becomes very
difficult to compare meaningfully the "intelligence" of a Western
white man with that of a Gurkha or a black. What we call intelligence is constructed with a large number of components having
wide human variability. Both heredity and environment play
important roles. Much of the nature vs. nurture controversy over
intelligence thus far has centered on arguments that suggest
that heredity is more important than environment.

The best evidence to support a genetic basis for intelligence
is the observation that the closer the family relationship the
greater the similarity of I.Q. scores. This becomes particularly
striking with identical twins, even if they are reared apart.[19]
From statistical analysis of this kind of data the estimate has been
made of a 75–85 per cent genetic component of I.Q. scores, while
15–25 per cent is ascribed to environmental causes. These claims
for the genetic determination of I.Q. are meant to apply to a

[18] F. W. Warburton, "The Ability of the Gurkha Recruit," *British Journal of Psychology* 42 (1951), pp. 123–33.
[19] L. Erlenmeyer-Kimling and L. F. Jarvik, "Genetics and Intelligence: a Review," *Science* 142 (1963), pp. 1477–79.

given population and not to any individual in that population. And these calculations are valid for that population at a given time and circumstance only. *There is no such thing as a universal genetic I.Q. determination, and we therefore cannot measure it for all people once and for all.*[20]

The most important conclusion to be drawn from this examination of data is that if the circumstances of testing change, the genetic contribution might be different also. There remain a number of major unresolved issues in the analysis of these data. For example, even when identical twins are reared separately, they are usually living in pretty much the same environment. There are only relatively rare circumstances under which one could imagine a significant upward or downward socioeconomic mobility among closely related family groups.

There is also the common but dangerous fallacy of making I.Q. scores synonymous with what we call intelligence. Dr. Arthur Jensen states that intelligence, like electricity, is easier to measure than to define. He also properly points out that "intelligence" should not be regarded as completely synonymous with "mental ability," which he defines as the totality of a person's mental capacity.[21] Thus I.Q. may reflect an important part, but only a part, of mental capacity, while only a segment of that part has an undefined genetic component. One of the best and most spectacular demonstrations of this is the peculiar kind of limited intelligence sometimes found in individuals known as *idiots savants*. These are individuals who can perform almost incredible feats of memory and mental calculation, yet are often of very low mental competence in almost every other aspect of intelligent behavior.

Dr. Florence Goodenough described a boy of twelve with a mental age of four who had a remarkable ability to mimic men

[20] R. M. C. Huntley, in *Genetic and Environmental Factors in Human Ability*, ed. by J. E. Mead and A. S. Parkes (New York: Plenum Press, 1966), p. 201.
[21] A. R. Jensen, "How Much Can We Boost I.Q. and Scholastic Achievement?" *Harvard Educational Review* 39 (1969), pp. 1–123.

and animals. He imitated a cat fight so true to life that stray cats within earshot rushed to the supposed scene of action. Dr. Goodenough also mentioned the case of Bertrand, a boy of twelve with a mental age of less than three, slurred and indistinct speech, the gait of an ape, and poor bladder control day and night. The simplest routine tasks of daily life were beyond his mastery. At a special school, while he made absolutely no progress at first, he became completely enthralled by such stories as "The Adventures of the Little Red Hen." Then, to the teacher's utter amazement, Bertrand would suddenly identify single words written on recognition cards and join the other children in reading lessons. By the end of the first year he could read anything that his limited understanding would permit—such books as *Peter Rabbit*. This phenomenal progress delighted Bertrand's parents, who supplied him with a prodigious number of infantile classics. Yet Bertrand made no progress at all in other endeavors. He still could not dress himself or control his bladder. He could not count to two, but always counted "one" or "more than one"; however, he could repeat numbers as far as 10, and read them to 100.

Goodenough also cites the story of the famous vaudeville stage exhibition of a feeble-minded boy, Blind Tom, early in this century. Like Bertrand, Blind Tom could not dress himself, but he could reproduce with mechanical accuracy even complex tunes after hearing them only once.[22]

One group of investigators describes a pair of identical twins who could determine in a fraction of a second the day of the week of any day of the year. One of the twins could do so over a range of more than six thousand years. The remarkable thing about these twins is that they had a subnormal I.Q., ranging around 65, and that neither of them could add or subtract even simple numbers.[23]

---

[22] F. L. Goodenough, *Mental Testing, Its History, Principles and Applications* (New York: Rinehart & Company, 1949), p. 350.
[23] W. A. Horowitz, C. Kestenbaum, E. Person, and L. Jarvik, "Identical Twins—*Idiots Savants*—Calendar Calculators," *American Journal of Psychology* 121 (1965), pp. 1075–79.

The performance of these *idiots savants* is a mystery. A small clue in the last case is that one twin found a perpetual calendar when he was six and spent many hours poring over it. This interest was shared by his brother years later. But how could this interest of two mentally retarded boys evolve into such an impressive ability to perform complex calculations? To this question posed of the twins, they could answer only, "It's in my head." Perhaps a photographic memory of the perpetual calendar itself was involved, as has been the case with many other *idiots savants*. But this still does not explain their ability to perform this amazing feat.

The *idiots savants* challenge our unanswered questions about the nature of intellectual processes, and are a monument to our ignorance on the subject. Until this challenge is overcome it will be premature to draw final conclusions about the structure and meaning of intelligence, and to prematurely assign an overwhelming hereditary contribution to the expression of intelligence.

Chapter VII

FROM BREAST TO GRUEL

Kwashiorkor is a widespread form of infant malnutrition. Its strange name was introduced to the medical profession by Dr. Cicerly D. Williams, who learned it from the Accra people of what is now the Republic of Ghana, where the disease is prevalent.[1]

The African word "kwashiorkor" means the disease an infant gets when his mother displaces him from her breast for a newborn infant. When this happens, usually between nine months and one year of age, the deposed infant is denied his mother's milk without receiving an adequate dietary replacement. The substitute is often gruel, which is deficient in essential amino acids. An infant being fed at its mother's breast is healthy and full of vitality. But when it is abruptly switched to, say, a diet of cornmeal gruel, its feet, legs, and, later, other parts of the body swell.[2] Vomiting and diarrhea follow. Skin and hair sometimes lose their pigmentation, resulting in discolored stripes of hair.[3]

---

[1] C. D. Williams, "Kwashiorkor: A Nutritional Disease of Children Associated with a Maize Diet," *Lancet* 229 (1935), p. 1151.
[2] C. D. Williams, "A Nutritional Disease of Childhood Associated with a Maize Diet," *Archives of Disease in Childhood* 8 (1933), p. 423.
[3] M. Autret and M. Béhar, "Le Syndrome de Polycarence de l'Enfance en Amérique Centrale (Kwashiorkor)," *Bulletin de l'Organisation Mondiale de la Santé* 11 (1954), p. 891.

Behavior also changes. Kwashiorkor victims are apathetic and peevish. In severe cases they are listless, with no interest in the world around them and unresponsive to stimuli, including food. When disturbed they are irritable and cry easily. The behavioral changes accompanying kwashiorkor have been abundantly documented, notably by the late Dr. Reginald F. A. Dean, Director of the Medical Research Council, Infantile Malnutrition Research Unit, Mulago Hospital, in Kampala, Uganda.

Superstition, ignorance, and tradition contribute to a denial of proper foods to the infant. These include the widespread custom of reserving the best protein foods, including milk, fish, and meat, for the elders, a prejudice against giving milk or eggs to infants, and the mistaken conviction that the best food for weaned infants includes maize gruel with sugar and perhaps the addition of a little bit of milk.

Customs related to weaning, however, have an important survival value. They are passed on from generation to generation, and the life of the infant depends on their strict enforcement. In primitive societies protein-rich foods are often the carriers of fatal germ-borne diseases. People believe they can save lives by avoiding protein-rich foods such as milk. Mothers have become accustomed to withhold milk from infants after observing that it "causes" diseases that can kill their babies. The price paid for survival may be mental retardation. Centuries-old traditions can be changed only when sanitation conditions are improved.

Some societies prize cattle as symbols of wealth rather than for their milk. Others sell the milk to purchase high-caloric foods, as is done in the southeastern part of the United States. In some cases cow's milk is unsuitable for human consumption because of rinderpest or tuberculosis, or the animals produce little or no milk because of the shortage of suitable fodder. It is not generally appreciated that the effective utilization of milk requires a very high degree of technological competence, purchasing power, and sophistication.[4]

---

[4] G. G. Graham, "Effect of Infantile Nutrition on Growth," *Federation Proceedings* 26 (1967), pp. 139–43.

Milk must be collected under conditions that will preserve it as a food, in particular because it is such a good medium for the growth of microorganisms. It must be stored under cold, aseptic conditions unless it is drunk within a short time following collection, which greatly limits its usefulness. Longer-term storage and transportation beyond the immediate area of its production require refrigeration, pasteurization, condensation, or evaporation for canning. The know-how for these complex and expensive processes requires resources that are not available to poor or primitive peoples.

Kwashiorkor is a nutritional disease associated with gross protein deficiency coupled with excessive intake of carbohydrates. What complicates the clinical picture, however, is that kwashiorkor is almost always accompanied by other problems, particularly infectious diseases resulting from lowered resistance brought about by malnutrition.

Bad temper and constant whining are common among kwashiorkor victims. Doctors investigated the disease in the central province of the Belgian Congo and reported that "big psychological or nervous problems are not found among the ill . . . [but] apparently they have a mind somewhat less alert, a more pronounced apathy. Unquestionably, there is retardation if not total arrest of all intellectual development."[5]

Drs. Geber and Dean studied twenty-five young kwashiorkor victims who were brought with their mothers to the Mulago Hospital for treatment and observation. The history of these children followed the classic pattern; so long as breast feeding lasted, the infant grew normally. After about a year, the child was weaned to a diet that rarely contained any milk and consisted mainly of cooked bananas, sweet potatoes, and manioc, with sauces made from beans and ground nuts. While meat was served to the family once or twice a week, the young child

---

[5] M. Geber and R. F. A. Dean, "The Psychological Changes Accompanying Kwashiorkor," *Courrier* 6 (1956), p. 3. Quotation of Dr. G. Doucet translated from the original French by the author.

received nothing more of it than a little of the accompanying gravy. After a few months on this diet the symptoms of kwashiorkor appeared.

On admission to the hospital, severely ill children were apathetic except for monotonous crying for long periods, especially when disturbed for examination or treatment. This resentment of interference surprised the investigators by its unexpected violence. Most children could not be induced to take any nourishment other than a thin liquid. "[The child would sleep] relatively little and usually had his eyes fully open, looking at nothing."[6] Some mothers ignored the sick child until his condition improved. Then they became more interested. The relationship of mother to child was often broken. The history of thirteen out of the twenty-five children studied included earlier separation from the mother to live with a grandparent or other relative, in accordance with local custom.

The intense need of the child for his mother emphasized to Drs. Geber and Dean the *total* dependence of the child on his mother; to protect himself from loss of contact he had retreated into infantilism. Yet the mother usually did not respond to this overwhelming need and remained passive to the child's demand for her continuous concern, love, and attention. Thus malnutrition in general, and kwashiorkor in particular, being primarily a nutritional disease of the young infant, reap a harvest of inhumanity at the most elemental level of human relationships, that of a child to its mother, which is a relationship unique to mammals, reflecting the long-drawn-out process of full brain development.

Infant nutrition begins with milk. Apart from the striking dominance of the brain, mammals are characterized by the female's possession of milk-secreting organs, whose function is triggered by the process of birth. Milk provides for an automatic continuation of fetal growth outside the mother's body. This relationship among birth, lactation, and growth, characteristic of the

---

[6] Ibid., p. 7.

class of mammals, is most remarkable among the human species. In all other species the young must forage and fight for their own food from the moment of birth on. The brain of other mammals is considerably simpler and more limited in the scope of its performance than that of the human species, but it will reach maturity much sooner with far less vulnerability to environmental vagaries.

The number of mammary glands is related to the average size of the litter born to that species. The characteristics of the milk produced by them also closely match the requirements of the species. While it is possible to feed the milk of one species to another, as is the case with cow's milk for human beings, milk varies very widely in composition to meet the specific requirements of given species. Infant rats, for example, are immune to malaria, because rat milk is deficient in the compound para-aminobenzoic acid, which is essential for the development of malarial microorganisms in the bloodstream of the rat.[7] The reason for the resistance to malaria of human infants during the first six months of life in infested tropical areas may be that human milk is also deficient in para-aminobenzoic acid.[8]

There are also important practical advantages to human milk. It costs nothing, it is free of contaminants, its composition remains essentially constant, it has the right temperature, it is readily available on demand, and it provides an opportunity for tenderness and affection between mother and child.

There is a direct relationship between the rate of growth of an infant of a particular species and the amount of protein found in its mother's milk. A baby rat, for example, doubles its birth weight in six days and rat milk contains 12 per cent protein, a very large amount. A goat doubles its birth weight in fourteen days and the protein content of goat's milk is 6 per cent. A human infant doubles its birth weight in 180 days and human

---

[7] B. G. Maegraith, T. Deegan, and E. S. Jones, "Suppression of Malaria by Milk, *British Medical Journal* 2 (1952), p. 1382.

[8] F. Hawking, "Milk, p-aminobenzoate and Malaria of Rats and Monkeys," *British Medical Journal* 1 (1954), p. 425.

milk contains only 1.6 per cent protein. By contrast, cow's milk contains 3.8 per cent protein for a doubling rate of seventy days.[9]

In comparison with cow's milk, human milk contains a considerable amount of a substance called the "lactobacillus bifidus factor," named after a bacterium that grows readily in human milk. This factor may have important but as yet undefined properties needed by the growing infant.[10]

Human milk also contains factors that protect the infant against such diseases as scurvy, rickets, and anemia, and promote growth of the proper intestinal bacterial flora. The composition of human milk may even be specifically related to the rapid growth of the brain.[11]

Biochemical investigators of milk are uncovering new and unsuspected differences between human and cow's milk that may prove to be important. For example, human milk contains 7 per cent linoleic acid, a lipid component, while cow's milk contains practically none. There are also significant differences in calcium and phosphorus-salt content. Babies fed cow's milk have been found to have more nitrogen, calcium, and phosphorus in their bodies than those fed human milk.[12]

The affluent middle class of the Western world takes it for granted that modern technology has contributed beneficially to the quality of life. In fact technology has worsened life for poor populations. It has destroyed centuries-old practices that served as an adequate balance for the community's needs. In the new vacuum, little has been devised to take their place.

Among the world's underprivileged peoples, advancing technology has exacerbated an already dire situation, particularly

[9] B. S. Platt and A. Moncrieff, "Nutritional Comparison of Human and Cow's Milk for Infant Feeding," *British Medical Bulletin* 5 (1947), p. 177.

[10] P. György, "A Hitherto Unrecognized Biochemical Difference Between Human Milk and Cow's Milk," *Pediatrics* 11 (1953), p. 98.

[11] H. K. Waller, "The Importance of Breast Feeding," *British Journal of Nutrition* 6 (1952), p. 210.

[12] H. Bakwin, "Infant Feeding," *Journal of Clinical Nutrition* 1 (1953), p. 349.

with regard to malnutrition. Although the severity of this situation has probably not changed much, its character has undergone a subtle but enormously important shift. Malnutrition now strikes children at an increasingly earlier age, and therefore the proportion of children with possible mental deficiencies is growing.

This is because as more countries enter the technological race and begin to industrialize, breast feeding by mothers has decreased precipitously; their infants, usually born in the hovels of burgeoning urban areas, therefore face malnutrition in the early months of life with increasing frequency. In Chile, one of the most rapidly developing nations of the world, women have abandoned breast feeding, and infant mortality has climbed to one of the highest rates in South America.[13] Even though the mortality rate is extremely high, the vast majority of these malnourished infants survive, with all the potential mental and physical consequences of malnutrition. Similar conditions exist in the urban slums and the backward rural areas of major industrial nations, including the United States.

In 1963 Drs. M. B. Stoch and P. M. Smythe of the Department of Child Health, Red Cross Memorial Children's Hospital and University of Cape Town, South Africa, published a now widely quoted report of a five-year research project involving forty-two children, entitled "Does Undernutrition During Infancy Inhibit Brain Growth and Subsequent Intellectual Development?" They concluded that it does, and wrote that their findings "are certainly suggestive that severe and prolonged undernutrition during infancy can permanently retard brain growth and intellectual development and, if confirmed, they add much emphasis and urgency to the need for good nutrition at this age."[14]

The investigation of Drs. Stoch and Smythe involved the study

---

[13] M. Winick, "Malnutrition and Brain Development," *Journal of Pediatrics* 74 (1969), pp. 667–69.
[14] M. B. Stoch and P. M. Smythe, "Does Undernutrition During Infancy Inhibit Brain Growth and Subsequent Intellectual Development?" *Archives of Diseases in Childhood* 38 (1963), pp. 546–52.

of two groups of twenty-one "Cape Coloured"* children between the ages of ten months and three years, for a period of five years. The difference between these two groups of children was the state of their nutrition. One half came from malnourished families, while the other half, as closely matched as possible in all other respects, came from families with stable income and adequate nutrition. All the children were given thorough physical and psychological examinations on a regular basis. The results of these examinations, including height, weight, and head circumference (which can be correlated with brain weight) all favored the adequately fed group.

Some of the ascription of significance to these and other similar observations has been severely criticized by a number of investigators in the field, particularly Dr. Rose E. Frisch of the Harvard University Center for Population Studies.[15] Dr. Frisch rightly points out that much of the evidence for a relationship between malnutrition and permanent mental retardation is at best indirect, and that many other factors, including that of social impoverishment, may be at least as important as nutrition. While strong arguments can be raised against attributing deficient height, weight, or head circumference solely to malnutrition, these observations, reported by Drs. Stoch and Smythe among others, are consistent with the finding of malnutrition. Particularly striking was the large mean-I.Q. difference between the malnourished and adequately fed groups of children: 70.86 for the first, compared with 93.48 for the second, a mean difference of more than twenty-two points.†

---

* "Cape Coloured," according to Webster's Third New International Dictionary, is "a native or inhabitant of So. Africa of mixed European and African or Malayan descent." This is the largest of the racially mixed peoples of South Africa and is socially intermediate between Europeans and Negroes.
[15] R. E. Frisch, "Does Malnutrition Cause Permanent Mental Retardation in Human Beings?" *Psychiatria, Neurologia, Neurochirurgia* 74 (1971), pp. 463–79.
† This mean difference was calculated to be significant at a probability level less than 1%. That is, there is only one chance in one hundred that this result could be due to pure chance. Hence there is a 99% probability that the researcher's hypothesis is correct.

Another early study of the effects of infant malnutrition on mental development that has received considerable attention is that of Drs. Vera Cabak and R. Najdanvic of the Pediatric Clinic of Sarajevo, Yugoslavia.[16] Children selected for this study were admitted to the Hospital for Sick Children in Sarajevo between 1951 and 1957 after a diagnosis of malnutrition. These children were at that time between the ages of four and twenty-four months, and were 27 per cent or more below the normal average weight for their age. Children suffering from clearly recognized diseases such as tuberculosis or central-nervous-system problems were excluded from the study.

This was a retrospective study, that is, one in which early records were examined years later. In this case the children were between seven and fourteen years of age at the time of the investigation. The parents of these children were mainly unskilled or skilled laborers, but one third were professionals or military officers. While this work suffers from serious deficiencies, particularly the lack of an adequately selected control group, it adds its weight to the total burden of indirect evidence. Of the thirty-six malnourished children tested, only half were within the normal I.Q. range, and twelve of them had a recorded I.Q. of 70 or lower. Their average I.Q. was 88, while that of other Serbian children from a similar environment was 105.

An explanation is needed here for use of the term "control group" above in leveling criticism at the study of Drs. Cabak and Najdanvic. The concept of control is paramount in all scientific work. Most scientific experiments require that a distinction be made between two related circumstances, one of which serves as the standard of comparison while the other is the experimental condition. Unless such a comparison can be made, it is not possible to identify a difference which may be caused by the experimental conditions.

It is through well-conceived and elegantly designed experi-

---

[16] V. Cabak and R. Najdanvic, "Effect of Undernutrition in Early Life on Physical and Mental Development," *Archives of Diseases in Childhood* 40 (1965), pp. 532–34.

ments that scientific advances are made. Many of these experiments involve comparisons that reveal unexpected differences. When adequate "control groups" are used, it is possible to detect early differences and to pinpoint the precise cause of this difference. The talent of a scientist is best demonstrated by the skill and ingenuity he uses in the conception and execution of experiments that contribute significantly to scientific knowledge. The ability to devise experiments with meaningful controls requires long and arduous training and represents the foundation of experimental work.

This control requirement poses a particularly difficult, if not presently insoluble, problem in relating malnutrition directly to brain development and subsequent mental performance. Human controls cannot be selected and regulated as can caged laboratory animals, and even standardized laboratory animals exhibit wide variations, which tend to cloud the significance of observations on them. Thus in their selection of "control groups" of adequately fed children to compare with the malnourished "experimental groups," Drs. Stoch and Smythe, Drs. Cabak and Najdanvic, and all other investigators in this extraordinarily complex field face almost insurmountable human obstacles in their search for clear-cut and definitive answers to the problem.

Until a scientist of genius identifies a more direct approach, probably of a biochemical nature, the best that can be done is to adjust to compromises and employ the powerful discipline of statistical analysis to the compromised results. This means drawing conclusions based on the probability of their being correct.

In the ever-lengthening chain of evidence linking malnutrition to stunted brain development, Drs. Myron Winick and Pedro Rosso of the Department of Pediatrics, Cornell University Medical College, in New York, have provided valuable information on the direct effect of early malnutrition on the brain itself.[17]

---

[17] M. Winick and P. Rosso, "The Effects of Severe Early Malnutrition on Cellular Growth of the Human Brain," *Pediatric Research* 3 (1969), pp. 181–84.

They obtained nineteen brains from Santiago, Chile, of children
who died accidentally. Ten of these brains were from well-
nourished Chilean children and nine were from children severely
malnourished during their first year of life. Drs. Winick and
Rosso analyzed weight and protein content, and determined
brain-cell numbers by using the method described in Chapter
III. They also compared these data with similar data on normal
children in the United States. They found that the brains of well-
nourished Chilean children contained the same number of cells
as those of well-nourished U.S. children.

By contrast, the brains of all nine of the severely malnourished
Chilean children contained a drastically lower number of brain
cells. The younger the children were when malnutrition struck
them, the more drastic was the reduction in brain-cell number.
Three of these malnourished children, who weighed less than
2,000 grams (4.4 lbs.) at birth, had a 60 per cent reduction in
brain-cell number. Drs. Winick and Rosso, however, cautioned
that they were not able to determine whether this astounding
reduction in the normal number of brain cells was due to intrauterine or to early postnatal malnutrition.

These investigators also demonstrated that during the first
months of life, the reduced head circumference in malnourished
children reflected accurately the reduced number of cells as well
as the reduced lipid content of the brain.[18] This was done by
studying in Santiago, Chile, ten brains taken either from fetuses
(the products of therapeutic abortions) or from children who
had died by accident or poisoning. In the study of prehistoric
man recounted in Chapter II, brain size was estimated from skull
volume, which is a better measurement than head circumference.
Since skull volume cannot be directly determined in living children, head circumference can be used with a fair degree of
accuracy to determine brain size.

Continuing these studies, Dr. Winick and his collaborators
made other important investigations. They examined thirty-one

---

[18] M. Winick and P. Rosso, "Head Circumference and Cellular Growth of
the Brain in Normal and Marasmic Children," *Journal of Pediatrics* 74
(1969), p. 774.

brains from humans ranging in age from a thirteen-week-old fetus to a thirteen-month-old infant, and demonstrated that new brain cells (probably all neuroglia) formed until the infant reached the age of about five months. Thereafter, continued growth was the result of accumulation of proteins and other substances, including perhaps lipids, rather than addition of new cells.[19] Thus these studies emphasized the importance of postnatal nutrition, and conversely the risks to which an infant may be exposed by malnutrition during this period.

But all significant growth in an infant's brain does not stop at the age of five months. Drs. Winick, Rosso, and John Waterlow also examined the brains from twenty-eight children up to two years of age from Santiago, Chile, and from Jamaica, West Indies.[20] Twelve of these brains were from well-nourished children, while the other sixteen were from severely malnourished children exhibiting emaciation and reduced head circumference at the time of death. Each brain was dissected into three major anatomical parts and analyzed by standard biochemical methods. The key findings were these: there is a major progressive increase in weight and protein content in all parts of the brain during the first two years of life; the brain weight increases 7 *times*, while that of its proteins increases 12 *times*, between birth and two years of age; among the brains of severely malnourished children there were strikingly lower weights and protein content at comparable ages.

This study also confirmed the earlier observations that brain cells increase rapidly in number only during the early months of life and more slowly thereafter until about one year of age, at which time very few additional cells are produced. All increases in weight thereafter involve increasing cell volume, protein content, and lipid content rather than the production of new cells, thus confirming the results of the other studies.

---

[19] M. Winick, "Changes in Nucleic Acid and Protein Content of the Human Brain During Growth," *Pediatric Research* 2 (1968), pp. 352–55.
[20] M. Winick, P. Rosso, and J. Waterlow, "Cellular Growth of Cerebrum, Cerebellum and Brain Stem in Normal and Marasmic Children," *Experimental Neurology* 26 (1970), pp. 393–400.

Marasmus is the type of malnutrition suffered by the children whose brains Dr. Winick and his team studied. It is far more damaging to early brain development than kwashiorkor. Marasmus is primarily the result of chronic malnutrition arising from a simple insufficiency of food, and thus from a shortage of calories. The U. S. National Research Council Food and Nutrition Board has established that infants should have 110 calories per kilogram (2.2 lbs.) of body weight per day in the first year of life and 1,200 calories per day thereafter until age 3.[21] A child suffering from a grossly calorie-deficient diet is severely underweight, with the facial appearance of a wizened old person somewhat resembling a monkey, and "flaky-paint" skin patches, but with normal hair and little of the tissue swelling characteristic of kwashiorkor.

Marasmus results from near starvation, and generally develops during the first year of life in infants whose diet is very low in both calories and protein. Kwashiorkor usually develops after the first year, though it is frequently found earlier. A child suffering from marasmus is alert and has a good appetite, in contrast to one suffering from kwashiorkor. In marasmus the amino-acid balance is normal, while in kwashiorkor the amino-acid balance in the blood is disturbed and exhibits deficits of certain blood proteins. In preindustrial societies, infants have been protected from marasmus, because the custom of breast feeding until at least six months of age has been widespread.[22] But as this practice has declined,[23] the risks of mental retardation may be rising.[24]

---

[21] U. S. National Research Council, Food and Nutrition Board, *Recommended Dietary Allowances*, NRC Reprint and Circular Series No. 129 (Washington: National Research Council, 1948).

[22] N. S. Scrimshaw and M. Béhar, "Malnutrition in Underdeveloped Countries," *New England Journal of Medicine* 27 (1965), pp. 137 and 193.

[23] F. Monckeberg, "Effect of Early Marasmic Malnutrition on Subsequent Physical and Psychological Development," in *Malnutrition, Learning and Behavior*, N. S. Scrimshaw and J. E. Gordon, eds. (Cambridge, Mass.: MIT Press, 1968), p. 269.

[24] F. Monckeberg, "Malnutrition and Mental Behavior," *Nutrition Reviews* 27 (1969), p. 191.

Marasmus is a chronic disease found among infants in the slums of industrial societies. It is caused by malnutrition arising from early weaning followed by a calorie-deficient substitute for breast milk. By contrast, kwashiorkor is an acute disease of infants in underdeveloped countries, usually found among older children whose breast feeding is prolonged beyond the first year.[25] The terms kwashiorkor and marasmus correspond to two different clinical syndromes whose presence depends upon a variety of factors including: age of the child; age at weaning; type, nutritive value, and quantity of food taken; as well as the nature and severity of infectious diseases accompanying these conditions. But in practice, since both forms of malnutrition are frequently found together in varying degrees of severity, scientists working in the field have adopted the term protein-calorie malnutrition to describe the frequently found combination of these two clinical conditions.

The effects of early marasmus malnutrition on the child's physical and mental development after recovery have been studied by Dr. Fernando Monckeberg of the University of Chile at Santiago, Chile.[26] As we have seen, malnutrition in a rapidly industrializing country begins at an early age because of the dramatic decrease in breast feeding that usually accompanies industrialization. When this change is superimposed upon poor social, economic and sanitary conditions, bottle feeding is not a satisfactory substitute for the mother's breast.[27] Under these conditions children sicken, and those who are admitted to the hospital frequently weigh not much more at six or seven

[25] R. E. Klein, J. P. Habicht, and C. Yarbrough, "Effects of Protein-Calorie Malnutrition on Mental Development," *Advances in Pediatrics* 18 (1971), pp. 75–91.

[26] F. Monckeberg, "Effect of Early Marasmic Malnutrition on Subsequent Physical and Psychological Development," in *Malnutrition, Learning and Behavior*, N. S. Scrimshaw and J. E. Gordon, eds. (Cambridge, Mass.: MIT Press, 1968), p. 269.

[27] F. Monckeberg, *Programs for Combatting Malnutrition in the Pre-school Child in Chile* (Washington: National Academy of Sciences-National Research Council, 1966), p. 74.

months of age than they did at birth. Many of them die, even
with good hospital care and treatment.

Fourteen such children were admitted to Dr. Monckeberg's
hospital metabolic ward. Five of these were male and nine female. The mean weight on admission was 3.3 kilograms (7 lb.
4 oz.), and the onset of marasmus had occurred between one
and five months of age. They were treated for long periods, then
discharged with an assured supply of 20 liters (5½ gal.) of fresh
milk per month. Similar amounts of milk were provided for all
other preschool children in the family to insure that none of the
milk supply would be diverted to favor one of the other children.

All the discharged children were kept under regular medical
surveillance for many years through visits to the out-patient department of the hospital. When these children reached the age
of three to six years, all appeared to have fully recovered from
their early marasmic malnutrition and were found to be clinically
normal. Their biochemical index of nutrition, that is to say their
blood hemoglobin, hematocrit, total protein, and albumin were
all within normal limits. But their height and weight were not
normal. Weight was above and height below those values considered normal for children of the ages at which they were measured. The appearance, therefore, was that of obese children.
The head circumference, a measure of brain size, was in all fourteen cases below normal, and in four of the children drastically
so. The average I.Q. of these children was 62, and the highest 76.

Of all other tests, the most revealing was the test for language
ability, which showed the greatest lag for malnourished children.
Dr. Monckeberg, of course, could not swear that these children
did in fact drink all the milk provided them during these years,
but results of periodic medical examinations, as well as performance on the biomedical index of nutrition, indicated that they
did maintain good nutrition during the years following recovery
from early-life marasmus. Dr. Monckeberg concluded that brain
damage sustained in infancy as a result of marasmic malnutrition
persists at least through the sixth year of life in spite of improved
nutritional circumstances. The average intelligence quotient of

these children, then, was significantly lower than that of the average Chilean preschool children from the same low socioeconomic background.‡

Of all studies of postnatal malnutrition and its possible influence on mental development, none has been more carefully conceived and carried out and on a grander scale than that of Dr. Joaquín Cravioto, Scientific Research Division, Hospital del Niño (IMAN) in Mexico City, together with several colleagues, in particular Dr. Elsa R. DeLicardie of Guatemala, and Dr. Herbert G. Birch, Department of Pediatrics, Albert Einstein College of Medicine, New York.[28] Dr. Cravioto and his team selected a small village in Guatemala to study. They defined children afflicted with early-life malnutrition as those between the ages of six and eleven who showed significantly smaller stature than their age mates. This definition is open to criticism because some of these children might have had small stature for reasons other than malnutrition, but it was the best choice under the circumstances. On a statistical basis, the assumption that these children were the most likely to have been malnourished proved to be a valid one, as will be seen later.

The presumed most-malnourished children selected were the shortest 25 per cent of the children in the village. Their performance was compared with that of the tallest 25 per cent. The tallest children were assumed to be those who had the least likelihood of having been malnourished, all other factors being equal. In this way it was possible to compare children with a common ethnic background and environment. In order to eliminate non-nutrition-related variables that might affect the children's stature, a careful analysis of other factors was made. This included:

1. Hereditary factor, which is the effect of parental stature on that of their children.

---

‡ For a probability factor of less than .1%, a very high statistical level of significance.

28 J. Cravioto, E. R. DeLicardie, and H. G. Birch, "Nutrition, Growth and Neurointegrative Development: An Experimental and Ecologic Study," *Pediatrics* 38 (1966), Supplement Part II, pp. 319–72.

2. General maturation lag, which was defined as a general slowing down of both physical and psychological processes related not to nutrition but to other factors such as hormonal malfunction.

3. Environmental influence on mental development. The social, economic, and educational status of the child's family have been shown to have an important influence on mental development.

These three variables were assessed and correlated, by taking complete and accurate records of all background information, before any conclusions were drawn. A copy of the comprehensive form used to collect these data was printed as an eight-page appendix to the report and included such details as: age, sex, occupation, and hereditary background of all family members including relatives or servants living in the household; ethnic group, religion, and language of all family members; housing details such as orientation of entrance, number of windows per room, electrification, and water; sanitary conditions such as toilet, bath, kitchen, and garbage facilities; family animals and quarters (inside or outside the house), handling of manure, and insects present; family gathering place and conditions of crowding and storage; personal hygiene habits of family members; literacy and use of printed information, radio, and television; family expenditures; family's own food production and use.

To assess the causal relationship of general maturation lag to stature and to overcome the possible effects of other environmental variables, a second sample of children of the same age, who had little likelihood of ever having been malnourished, was selected for comparison.

The investigators carefully considered the kind of test that would best determine the mental development of these children. They selected analyses of intersensory organization, which deal with the ability to use the basic five senses in an effectively coordinated manner. A great deal of accumulated scientific evidence on the subject was cited by Dr. Cravioto's team to support its choice. Intersensory integration is an essential part of man's ability to adapt and respond to his environment and is thus closely linked to the acquisition of cognitive skills. Dr. Cravioto in his report quotes the great English neurophysiologist and Nobel laureate Sir Charles Sherrington (1857–1952), the discoverer of nerve-cell function, in arguing about man's limited five senses, as saying, "The naive would have expected evolution in its course to have supplied us with more various sense organs for ampler perception of the world. . . . The policy has rather been to bring by the nervous system the so-called "five" into closer touch with one another. . . . A central clearing house of sense has grown up. . . . Not new senses, but better liaison between old senses, is what the developing nervous system has in this respect stood for."[29]

It is man's unique mental ability to coordinate the "five" senses that has given him the evolutionary edge. For example, the migration of the eyes to a common plane made stereoscopic vision possible, and integration of this new ability with manual dexterity gave man an unbeatable advantage in evolutionary selection. That integration was a crucial function, which the human brain was called upon to perform. Similarly, the four stages of human mental development defined by Piaget represent an increasingly sophisticated integration of the senses. The most exquisitely complex intersensory integration is involved in the processes of reading, writing, and speaking, achievements that so far are beyond the mental capacity of the most advanced primates below man.

Man interacts with the world around him through his classic and severely limited senses. But by remarkable coordination among them he is able to transcend these limitations and vastly expand his consciousness of the universe. This he does through the intervention of his brain. But unless man's brain is functioning properly, the high level of intersensory integration of which he is capable eludes him, reducing his appreciation of the environment to the limited scope of his separate "five" senses. Thus

<hr>

[29] J. Cravioto, E. R. DeLicardie, and H. G. Birch, "Nutrition, Growth and Neurointegrative Development: An Experimental and Ecologic Study," *Pediatrics* 38 (1966), Supplement Part II, pp. 319–72.

intersensory integration is a sensitive and meaningful measure of mental potential, especially among young children.[30]

The village of Magdalena, in which the study by Dr. Cravioto's team was carried out, is in the Department of Sacatepéquez, in the central zone of the Republic of Guatemala. It is about twenty-two miles from Guatemala City, the capital. The altitude of the village is 2,060 meters (6,580 ft.) above sea level. The climate is characterized by two clearly defined seasons, popularly called "summer," which is dry, and "winter," when heavy rains fall.

The population of Magdalena, more than 80 per cent Indian, consisted at that time of 1,620 persons, 323 of them children below the age of five, living in 333 families. Health conditions in the village had undergone a progressive change since the turn of the century. In the period 1901–5, for instance, the mortality rate was 43 per 1,000, while between 1958 and 1962 it had dropped to 15 per 1,000. Yet the death rate for infants below one year of age had remained unchanged at about 13 per cent, while between the ages of six and twelve it amounted to 2.8 per cent of the total deaths from 1958 to 1962. The main causes of death were diarrhea, measles, "worms," and "dropsy," in that order. The birth rate had been stationary at around 44 births per 1,000 since about 1950.

The villagers of Magdalena were small farmers who grew a variety of staples, primarily vegetables such as beans, lettuce, cabbage, carrots, and green peppers, and flowers for commercial purposes. The main commercial interchange was with the city of Antigua, serviced twice a week by bus, and with the capital by daily bus service. Although the diet had improved somewhat during recent years, mainly through increased consumption of milk products, greens, bananas, grains, roots, and fats, it remained significantly poor in proteins; even so, in this respect it was more adequate at the time of the study than it had been thirteen years previously.

---

[30] H. G. Birch and A. Lefford, "Two Strategies for Studying Perception in 'Brain-damaged' Children," in Brain Damage in Children: Biological and Social Aspects, H. G. Birch, ed. (Baltimore: Williams & Wilkins, 1963), p. 46.

The tallest 25 per cent and the shortest 25 per cent of the children in Magdalena were selected for study. These two groups comprised 143 children. Their socioeconomic environment was then subjected to the detailed analysis posed by the questions listed in the elaborate, eight-page questionnaire. The urban comparison group consisted of 120 children attending a private school whose pupils were drawn from upper-middle-class to upper-class families, all with high income and high educational backgrounds.

The tests for intersensory integration were simple and effective. Three different sensory classes were chosen for study. These were the visual, haptic, and kinesthetic modes. Visual involves recognition by sight. Haptic stands for the sensory perception obtained by active manual exploration of a test object. A blind person, for instance, will identify an object by feeling it with his hands. The kinesthetic sense is a passive one in which perception arises from muscle tension. In this instance, the kinesthetic sense from the wrist, elbow, and shoulder muscles was tested. The examiner did this by holding the child's arm behind a curtain and moving it in a circular, square, triangular, or other shape and having the child identify the shape by the perception obtained from these passive movements.

Eight geometric forms about 4 x 5 inches in size, consisting of circle, square, triangle, semicircle, hexagon, cross, diamond, and star, were used for these tests. Rigidly defined procedures were devised to standardize the test conditions. Three sets of paired interactions between visual, haptic, and kinesthetic senses were explored. They were the visual-haptic, visual-kinesthetic, and haptic-kinesthetic combinations. The children were tested individually in a quiet room, alone with the examiner. Each child was told beforehand what would happen. For example, in the visual-haptic pair he was told: "In this next game, I am going to show you a form like this circle. Then I am going to move your hand around like this. You are to tell me whether the shape your hand moves around is the same as the shape you see in front of you. To make the game more interesting, I am not going to let you see which shape your hand is going to go around. I will hold your hand behind this screen. You are not to look. We will do it like this."[31]

When the child understood the test, he was asked to judge whether the forms in front of him and behind the curtain were "the same" or "different." The number of correct and erroneous answers would then be recorded and compared. The results of these simple, but probing, tests were remarkable in their consistency. In all three series of paired tests, the tallest children of the rural village of Magdalena achieved the best scores, making significantly fewer errors than the shortest children. The urban children from the private school, however, obtained consistently better results than even the tallest children of Magdalena, regardless of their physical stature.

In some of the tests the differences in scoring were striking. In the visual-kinesthetic series, for instance, the tallest rural children made half as many errors, on the average, as the shortest rural children of the same age. The differences among the six-year-old children, youngest of those tested, were the greatest in several of the test series, these differences diminishing somewhat with increasing age. The fact that the private-school children did not show differences in performance associated with height is also very important. It suggests that differences in stature among well-nourished children arise primarily from heredity, unaffected by nutrition, and that this variable cannot be associated with mental capacity.

Assessment of the effect of heredity on the stature of the rural children of Magdalena was a very important part of the whole study. The statistical evaluation of this factor was carefully carried out by using extensive records obtained from the families of the children tested. *This examination failed to disclose any meaningful relationship between the height of the children and that of their parents.* This was an extremely important observation. It suggested that the existing influence of heredity on height

---

[31] J. Cravioto, E. R. DeLicardie, and H. G. Birch, "Nutrition, Growth and Neurointegrative Development: An Experimental and Ecologic Study," *Pediatrics* 38 (1966), Supplement Part II, p. 340. Quoted by permission.

was greatly overshadowed by the far more drastic influence of malnutrition. When malnutrition was *not* a factor, however, the hereditary component controlling height could be recognized. The investigators reported that there was a small but significant relationship between the height of an urban father and his private-school child, but none could be found between urban mother and child.

Other evidence for the importance of diet on stature is abundant. Stature has increased in the United States during the past century. In Japan it has increased strikingly since World War II, with increased prosperity and better diet. The small stature of some populations is thought to be genetically determined, when in fact it may result from dietary insufficiency in early life. When these populations make giant strides in their economic development and dietary status, as have the Japanese, their suddenly increased stature outstrips their supposed genetic potential.

A study by Dr. George G. Graham of the Department of Pediatrics, Johns Hopkins School of Medicine, Baltimore,[32] working at the British-American Hospital in Lima, Peru, emphasized the importance of diet on growth. In a thirty-four-month study of fifty-three malnourished infants and children, Dr. Graham was able to provide evidence that suggested that height, weight, and head-circumference deficits associated with early-life malnutrition could be improved by a good diet but could not be made up later, and that most of these children would be permanently stunted.

Some research workers caution that this increased stature could be due in part to a genetic selection of taller individuals, which under the negative influence of a hostile environment could favor for survival shorter individuals having smaller dietary requirements. The evidence, however, does not permit a determination of whether this is a significant factor.

Dr. Cravioto and his team also observed that the pattern of change in the test performance of the children as a function of

---

[32] G. G. Graham, "Effect of Malnutrition on Growth," *Federation Proceedings* 26 (1967), pp. 139–43.

increasing age was remarkably similar for all children tested, both rural and urban. The difference was that in achieving intersensory integration at a given age, the shortest lagged behind the tallest rural children, while urban children of all heights invariably were ahead of all rural children.

Since the height of the father in the urban-private-school group was found to be related to the height of his child, Dr. Cravioto's team decided to find out whether the father's height made any significant contribution to his child's intersensory test performance. The results of this examination showed that no significant relationship could be found between the father's height and the child's intersensory competence, thus again suggesting that there was no obvious hereditary influence on the relationship of these traits.

The conclusions that can be drawn from this study are therefore of overriding significance in studying the relationship between malnutrition and cognition. Differences in growth of the rural children tested are most likely to have arisen from the environment in which they were born and raised rather than from inherited causes. The environmental causes included infectious and parasitic diseases but predominantly focused on a diet chronically inadequate for growth, which predisposed the children to disease and greatly exacerbated the effects of malnutrition.[33]

One should not draw the conclusion from Dr. Cravioto's work that there is always a relationship between stature and intelligence. Only when early-life malnutrition is associated with reduced stature can this relationship be established. But even then the conclusion must be tempered by the influence of other factors, particularly that of social environment and sex differences on cognition.[34]

Nevertheless, the relationship among early-life malnutrition,

---

[33] D. Wilson, R. Bressani and N. S. Scrimshaw, "Infection and Nutritional Status. I. The Effect of Chicken Pox on Nitrogen Metabolism," *American Journal of Clinical Nutrition* 9 (1961), p. 154.

[34] R. E. Klein, J. Kagan, H. E. Freeman, C. Yarbrough, and J. P. Habicht, "Is Big Smart? The Relation of Growth to Cognition," *Journal of Health and Social Behavior* 13 (1972), pp. 219–25.

low stature, and lagging intersensory integration is a strongly suggestive one, though the exact nature of that relationship is yet to be fully defined. According to Dr. Cravioto's research group, at least two possibilities must be considered. The first alternative is that the poor socioeconomic conditions under which the child lives are responsible for two conditions of *independent* origin: one is poor intersensory integration, and the other is malnutrition, which is directly responsible for low stature. In this alternative, malnutrition and mental competence as measured by intersensory integration are related *only* by the fact that *both* arise from a poor environment.

The second alternative is that poor socioeconomic conditions are responsible for malnutrition *only*. Malnutrition, in turn, is a *direct* cause of *both* low stature *and* low mental competence as measured by intersensory integration.

Dr. Cravioto and his collaborators conclude that neither of these two alternative hypotheses can be rejected, but that a stronger case can be made for the second than for the first. The first alternative is based on the inference that social impoverishment, which includes inadequate opportunities for education, contributes directly to poor intersensory development. If this were true, low stature and poor intersensory integration would have been found to be uniformly associated with low family income and poor housing and sanitation, as well as a host of related factors.

The investigators in Magdalena, however, could find no such association, except for a positive correlation of the mother's educational level with intersensory adequacy of the child. This, of course, was to be expected because of the very close relationship of mother to child in the first years of life, during which the child belongs to the "women's world." But the lack of correlation found among poor intersensory development, low stature, and the household environment in which the child grew up is striking, and supports the hypothesis that malnutrition is directly related to poor intersensory integration.

In earlier chapters, we have discussed how malnutrition could *directly* affect brain development. The following three *indirect* consequences of malnutrition on intersensory development were also considered by Dr. Cravioto and his team:

1. Loss of learning time. Since a malnourished child is less responsive to his environment, he will have lost several months of living experience and therefore will lag behind normal children of the same age and environment.

2. Interference with learning during critical periods of development. Learning, like brain development, appears to take place in a defined sequence and schedule, as Piaget has shown. The so-called critical periods of learning, when delayed, omitted, or missed, may also be lost forever.[35]

3. Motivation and personality changes. The mother's response to an infant is to a great degree determined by the child's own vitality, as Drs. Geber and Dean, among many others, have so graphically shown. One of the first effects of malnutrition is apathy in the child, which then provokes apathy in the mother. This reduces drastically a child's interaction with his environment and isolates him from the world around him.

Mental development, of which intersensory integration represents a considerable part, is heavily dependent on this give-and-take with the environment and is the basis for learning, maturation, and interpersonal relations. Malnutrition-generated apathy, therefore, leads to a cumulative stimulus-response deficiency, which results in significant backwardness. The effects of this backwardness are felt most crushingly later on, when the child is faced with the increasingly complex learning tasks he must master to survive and prosper, especially in a technologically oriented society. Among these tasks is the ability to read and write. Reading and writing are most closely associated with the auditory-visual intersensory pair, and in a separate investigation Dr. Cravioto, in collaboration with Drs. Carlos E. Gaona and Herbert G. Birch, addressed himself specifically to an examina-

---

[35] J. P. Scott, "Critical Periods in Behavioral Development," *Science* 138 (1962), p. 949.

tion of the effect of early malnutrition on integration of that pair of senses.[36]

The subjects of this study were 296 children between seven and twelve years of age enrolled in the primary school of a rural village in southwestern Mexico. The experimental procedure used in Magdalena was also selected for this study. Integration of hearing and sight was tested by tapping out simple sounds and by exhibiting visual dot patterns on cards that corresponded to the sound patterns heard. Again the tallest children of all ages made significantly fewer errors in matching sound and sight patterns than did the shortest children of the same age, and both groups showed improved performance with increasing age. The greatest rate of improvement occurred between nine and eleven years of age, especially among the tallest children. Among the twelve-year-old children, 42 per cent of the tallest gave eight or more correct answers, 30 per cent of them achieving a perfect score. By contrast, only 9 per cent of the shorter children achieved a score of eight or more correct answers, with none making a perfect score.

In an earlier study led by Dr. Birch it was shown that retarded readers performed considerably less well in auditory-visual tests than normal readers.[37] Thus early-life malnutrition may be an important cause of damage to intersensory integration. This is often characterized later in the child's life by a pattern of failure, which begins in school and ends with maladaptation to society and lack of gainful employment.

Considerable controversy exists about the extent of recovery possible from severe early malnutrition. Some researchers claim that complete "catch-up" can take place.[38] The unanswered

[36] J. Cravioto, C. E. Gaona, and H. G. Birch, "Early Malnutrition and Auditory-Visual Integration in School-age Children," *Journal of Special Education* 2 (1967), pp. 75–82.

[37] H. G. Birch and L. Belmont, "Auditory-Visual Integration, Intelligence and Reading Ability in School Children," *Perceptual and Motor Skills* 20 (1965), pp. 295–305.

[38] J. S. Garrow and M. C. Pike, "The Long-term Prognosis of Severe Infantile Malnutrition," *Lancet* 1, 1967, p. 1.

question revolves around the problem of mental rather than physical "catch-up," and the evidence suggests that while a good physical recovery is possible, a good mental one is not. Among the studies focusing on this problem is the one undertaken by Drs. George G. Graham and Blanca Adrianzen T. of the Department of Pediatrics, School of Medicine, Johns Hopkins University, in co-operation with the Nutrition Research Institute of Lima, Peru.[39]

In this study eight severely malnourished infants and eight normal infants between seven and nine months of age were followed through a period of nine years of rehabilitation. The malnourished infants came from desperately poor families living in the slums surrounding the periphery of Lima, as they surround nearly all the large cities of the world, including Washington, D.C. These infants had been admitted to the British-American Hospital in that city. They lived in one-room shacks without flooring, windows, running water, sewage, electricity, or other amenities, and were born of a mother whose "spouse" was often unidentifiable, or chronically unemployed, and given to excessive drinking.

These seriously malnourished infants were able, when transferred to a much better home, to make rapid advances in growth and return to what the authors call "their genetically programmed size or very close to it." But they could make no such statement about the mental competence of these rehabilitated children as determined by I.Q. tests. All they could say was that there had been no mental improvement to parallel or match that observed in height and head size. The authors concluded with these words: "Of the many important factors responsible for measurable intelligence at eight years of age, certainly severe and prolonged deprivation during early life, whether at home or in an institution, looms as most impressive."[40]

---

[39] G. G. Graham and B. Adrianzen T., "Late 'Catch-up' Growth After Severe Infantile Malnutrition," *The Johns Hopkins Medical Journal* 131 (1972), pp. 204–11.
[40] Ibid., p. 211. Quoted by permission.

In a review of thirteen studies on the effect of severe early malnutrition on infant mental development, including a few discussed in this chapter, Drs. Joaquín Cravioto and Elsa R. DeLicardie concluded that severe nutritional deprivation at the time the central nervous system (which includes the brain) is growing rapidly may cause it measurable damage.[41] Particularly significant in this conclusion is the word "measurable." Whether the test used was an I.Q. test or an intersensory-integrative assessment, the results all pointed in the same direction. When compared to normal children, those who had a history of severe early malnutrition invariably scored significantly worse in these tests, with no evidence that complete recovery was possible.

That the ability to read, write, and speak involves intersensory perception can be readily demonstrated. For instance, the child's failure to respond adequately to the spatial orientation of a visual form can result in his inability to distinguish a number of letters in the alphabet that have the same shape but a different orientation. The lower case b, p, d, and q, and the capital letters N, Z, W, and M are frequent problems that any elementary-school teacher of disadvantaged children will cite as major stumbling blocks in learning to read. If such children find it difficult to recognize letters, the problem is compounded in having to write them down.

The influence of severe malnutrition on language development was also studied by Drs. DeLicardie and Cravioto by comparing nineteen malnourished children to a normal group of children of the same age. They were able to show that even after clinical recovery had taken place, a striking lag in language development remained with the malnourished children.[42] The ac-

---

[41] J. Cravioto and E. R. DeLicardie, "Mental Performance in School-age Children. Findings After Recovery from Early Severe Malnutrition," *American Journal of Diseases of Children* 120 (1970), pp. 404–10.

[42] E. R. DeLicardie and J. Cravioto, "Language Development in Survivors of Clinical Severe Malnutrition," unpublished manuscript (in press), courtesy of the authors.

cretion of knowledge available to the human species is denied such children. Over the years of dismal schooling, these deficiencies become cumulative, and the wherewithal of social and economic competition is permanently lost to them. Useless and unwanted, they often turn to antisocial behavior and crime to survive. They produce offspring whose deficiencies in turn condemn them to remain the flotsam and jetsam of civilization.

It is not yet established that malnutrition *causes* mental retardation, although it is clearly *associated* with it. Malnutrition seldom occurs as an isolated phenomenon. It is almost always found in an environment including poverty, ignorance, poor housing and sanitation, overcrowding, and a high prevalence of infectious and parasitic disease. These factors are associated with poor, illiterate, and, frequently, retarded parents. When such conditions exist, nutritional deficiencies are almost always found to coexist with deficiencies in intellectual stimulation. Any factor that plays an important role in bringing about malnutrition may also contribute to impaired mental development.

Based on these considerations, Drs. Michael C. Latham and Francisco Cobos of the Graduate School of Nutrition, Cornell University, and the Department of Nutrition, Harvard University, respectively, have proposed that the poor mental performance of malnourished children is due not to brain damage per se but rather to the fact that malnutrition has restricted the activities and learning opportunities of the child. These investigators point out that reduced activity is a protective response of the organism to conserve energy. A malnourished infant or child will appear passive, restrict his movements, greatly limit his time spent in play, and avoid verbalizing with his mother in order to save energy for essential needs, including growth. His subsequent poor performance in mental tests may be a consequence of the fact that he has been passively sitting around for much of his waking life.[43]

---

[43] M. C. Latham and F. Cobos, "The Effects of Malnutrition on Intellectual Development and Learning," *American Journal of Public Health* 61 (1971), pp. 1307–24.

This was recognized many years ago by Dr. Reginald F. A. Dean, who emphasized that a very early sign of recovery involves an improvement in interpersonal response. Said Dr. Dean, "The child who smiles is on the road to recovery."[44] These points were underscored by Dr. Herbert G. Birch, Department of Pediatrics, Yeshiva University, Albert Einstein College of Medicine, New York, in a report that reviews the relationship between malnutrition, learning, and intelligence. Dr. Birch states that it would be tragic to emphasize nutrition at the expense of other factors (social, cultural, educational, psychological) which also have an influence on intellectual development. What must be recognized is that within an all-encompassing effort to improve the conditions of disadvantaged populations, early-life nutritional considerations must occupy a prominent position.[45]

While a great deal of field research has been done on the consequences of severe early-life malnutrition, very little has been published on mild but chronic malnutrition or on the effects of malnutrition, of whatever degree of severity, persisting into the teens and later. Most malnourished infants remain malnourished throughout their lives, and what evidence is available suggests that the life span of their miserable existence is considerably foreshortened by lack of vitality and vulnerability to disease. Dr. Dean, in the last publication before his death, showed that even mild chronic malnutrition has demonstrable biochemical effects related to the growth of young children.[46] Future research is likely to uncover evidence establishing mild chronic malnutrition to be even more widespread than severe malnutrition, with nearly as serious consequences.

Finally we must confront the genetic considerations that apply to the mental capacity of disadvantaged peoples. The extent

[44] R. F. A. Dean, "The Effect of Malnutrition on the Growth of Young Children," *Bibliotheca Paediatrica* 72 (1960), pp. 111–22.

[45] H. G. Birch, "Malnutrition, Learning and Intelligence," *American Journal of Public Health* 62 (1972), pp. 773–83.

[46] R. F. A. Dean, "Effects of Malnutrition, Especially of Slight Degree, on the Growth of Young Children," *Courrier* 15 (1965), pp. 73–83.

of hereditary influence on mental development is a long way
from being resolved, but the following supports other evidence
in favor of a predominantly environmental influence on intelligence:

Investigations of disadvantaged populations have shown that
the motor coordination and intersensory adaptation of normal
newborn infants in these groups are equal to or better than those
used as the standard of comparison in the United States. They
include studies in Africa,[47,48] Guatemala,[49] and Mexico.[50,51]
Therefore the deficient mental performance of malnourished
children in these populations cannot have a dominant genetic
component, and must be ascribed to hostile environmental factors. A more thorough examination of the hereditary component
of the problem is made in the next chapter.

---

[47] S. Falade, *Contribution à une Étude sur le Développement de l'Enfant
d'Afrique Noire. Le Développement Psycho-moteur du Jeune Africain
Originaire du Sénégal au Cours de Sa Première Année.* (Paris: Foulon,
1955). (Thesis, University of Paris.)
[48] M. Geber and R. F. A. Dean, "The State of Development of Newborn
African Children," *Lancet* 1, 1957, pp. 1216–19.
[49] E. R. DeLicardie, H. G. Birch, and J. Cravioto, "Motor and Adaptive
Behavior in Newborn Guatemalan Infants," *Proc. Reunión Reglamentaria
Asociación de Investigación Pediátrica* (Cuautla, Morelia, Mexico, 1966).
[50] J. Cravioto, "Application of Newer Knowledge of Nutrition on Physical
and Mental Growth and Development," *American Journal of Public Health*
53 (1963), p. 1803.
[51] J. Cravioto *et al.*, "Motor and Adaptive Development of Premature Infants
from a Preindustrial Setting During the First Year of Life," *Biology of the
Neonate* 11 (1967), p. 151.

Chapter VIII

LIKE BEGETS LIKE:
GENETICS AND RACE

Seth Wright was a Massachusetts farmer with a problem. His farm, near the Charles River at Dover, was fenced by rough stones, a common sight in 1791, as it remains today, the familiar rural barrier of New England. Low stone fences meant that the lambs of his flock could easily jump over, and Seth Wright was losing too many of his lambs.

That year, a short-legged male lamb was born, the result of a spontaneous germinal mutation. By breeding the short-legged ram to his ewes, Wright obtained a few more short-legged lambs. By continuing to breed the short-legged sheep to each other, he eventually developed a line of short-legged sheep, which were unable to cross the low stone fence, thus neatly solving the problem and originating the Ancon breed of sheep. This was done from empirical experience, without knowledge of the principles governing heredity. Spontaneous mutations are an important part of the evolutionary concept, because they provide a basis for hereditary changes.

Since the dawn of man's appearance on this planet, he must have been conscious of the fact that like tends to beget only like. Oaks yield acorns, from which only oaks grow. Chicken eggs crack open to reveal only chicks. Dogs give birth to dogs only, and the same is true of every species of living thing. Not only does like beget like, but the close kinship between parents and progeny is governed by rigidly circumscribed natural laws. Family members resemble each other in physical characteristics such as size, shape, and color, as well as in some aspects of behavior.

History records widespread evidence for the application of this simple principle of like begets like. Agriculture was probably one of the first areas to be explored. The ancient Chinese selected empirically the most robust and highest-yielding rice plants to be propagated in their fields. In the Americas, maize breeding made it possible for this plant to become the staple food of the continent.

Maize* is native to America; there exists no evidence for its presence anywhere else in the world until after 1492. Through the technique of carbon dating, we can place the oldest maize found in South America at around 2,000 B.C. Archaeological specimens of maize found in New Mexico show that the early corn was being cultivated and improved through hybridization (cross-breeding) long before the coming of the white man. What makes maize such a fascinating subject for study is that it is probably the one cultivated plant whose enormous diversity exceeds that of all others. It is easily crossed with other maize to produce usually fertile species, and hybridization results in spectacular improvement in yield, size, taste, robustness, and variety. But a considerable problem in its propagation is that hybrid maize does not breed true; that is, it produces a whole gamut of different hybrids, which reflect all the characteristics of the parental strains rather than being limited to a single, clear-cut hybrid strain. The fact that the early inhabitants of the Americas were able to recognize this problem, and deal with it empirically and successfully, suggests that they had keen powers of observation, even though they had not the vaguest idea of the biological laws that govern the genetics of this plant.

---

* Maize is usually referred to as corn or Indian corn in the U.S.A. This is confusing because wheat is also called corn. We shall use the more specific term to avoid confusion.

Sir Francis Galton (1822–1911) was the first careful observer of human heredity, and he was also the first to introduce into his studies the powerful investigative tool of statistical analysis. His application of systematic techniques to biology was new, and it led to the publication, in 1869, of his classic work entitled *Hereditary Genius,* in which he proposed that illustrious persons beget other persons of note in all major areas of human endeavor. Galton supported his thesis by listing the pedigrees and their influence on race of the following prominent groups of men between 1660 and 1865: judges, statesmen, members of the peerage, military commanders, literary men, men of science, musicians, painters, divines (men of the church), and senior classics (professors) of Cambridge.

The puzzling addition to this list of oarsmen and wrestlers of the North Country is explained thus by Galton: "I propose to supplement what I have written about brain by two short chapters on muscle. No one doubts that muscle is hereditary in horses and dogs, but humankind are so blind to facts and so governed by preconceptions, that I have heard it frequently asserted that muscle is not hereditary in men. Oarsmen and wrestlers have maintained that their heroes spring up capriciously, so I have thought it advisable to make inquiries in the matter. The results I have obtained will beat down another place of refuge for those who insist that each man is an independent creation, and not a mere function, physically, morally, and intellectually, of ancestral qualities and external influences."[1]

Unfortunately, Galton was ignorant of the laws governing genetics. Furthermore, his impressive list of contemporary geniuses contained a substantial number of persons to whom posterity has not accorded the same degree of significance and importance it has to him.

Galton was a contemporary of the scientific genius Gregor Mendel, an Austrian monk whose classic experiments with peas represent the fundamental contribution that formed the basis of

---

[1] F. Galton, *Hereditary Genius,* An Inquiry into its Laws and Consequences (London: Macmillan & Co., 1969), p. 305.

modern genetics. Galton wrote his treatise at about the same time that Mendel studied peas, but neither of them knew of the existence of the other. Mendel published the results of his experiments in 1866, but they remained unrecognized until the turn of the twentieth century. Mendel himself probably never realized the full significance of his own discovery, and certainly few others did.

What Mendel did appears remarkably simple and straightforward; his success was due in part to his lucky (or inspired) choice of a suitable living organism, which made observation of single traits possible, and proper experimental conditions. He crossbred garden pea plants having certain readily identifiable traits, and noted the appearance of these traits in the progeny of these crosses. For example, he crossbred tall garden pea plants having gray-brown seeds with dwarf plants having white seeds, and observed the appearance of all these traits in the progeny. He noted that, contrary to expectation, this crossbreeding did not yield plants whose height was intermediate between the dwarf and the tall, but that he got only one or the other and nothing in between. He noted the same thing in the colors of the ripe seeds: they were either gray-brown or white, with none having an intermediate, grayish-pink color. In other words, the trait or *phenotype* was passed on intact in the hybrid progeny and was not a mixture of the traits found in the two parents. This finding, which embodies Mendel's first fundamental principle and which was called by him "purity of gamete," is of capital importance in understanding how heredity operates. *The potential for a given trait is passed on whole or not at all.* This is the first law of Mendelian genetics.

The next question was what determines whether or not the trait is passed on. Mendel observed that when he crossed a tall pea plant with a dwarf one, he obtained all tall progeny in the first generation and more tall progeny than dwarf in the second. A cross between a plant with gray-brown seeds and a plant with white seeds always yielded plants with only gray-brown seeds in the first generation, and more gray-brown than white-seeded

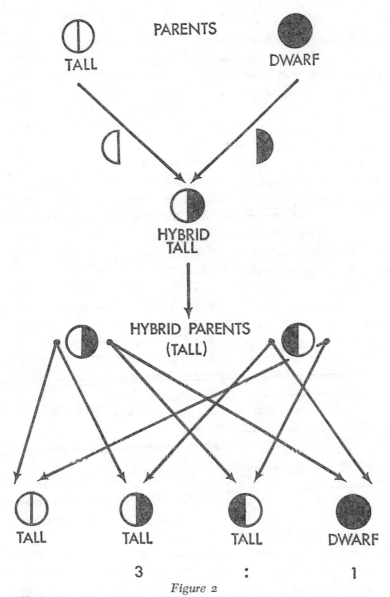

PARENTS

TALL

DWARF

HYBRID
TALL

HYBRID PARENTS
(TALL)

TALL   TALL   TALL   DWARF

3   :   1

Figure 2

Illustration of a cross between a tall and a dwarf pea plant (Mendel)
The TALL gene (white half circle) is dominant over the dwarf gene
(black half circle), and in the hybrid the phenotype will be TALL
(black & white). A cross between two hybrids will yield the familiar
3:1 ratio in the progeny because of the frequency of chance combinations of genes as is shown at the bottom of the illustration.

plants in the second generation. This was very puzzling to him, and he therefore carefully counted how many of each he obtained in the second generation. He noted that there were always roughly three times as many tall hybrids as dwarf ones, and also three times as many gray-brown-seeded plants as white-seeded ones. The simple cross between a tall and a dwarf garden pea plant is illustrated in Figure 2.

From these simple but laborious and time-consuming observations, Mendel deduced the second law of genetics. He figured out that in order to get a 3:1 ratio in the second generation there would have to be not *one* but *two* "gametes" controlling the appearance of a trait. This was a "flash of genius," a term characterized by a dramatically simple explanation of something that seems terribly complicated. Mendel arrived at the correct conclusion first by carefully counting the number of plants exhibiting each trait in the progeny, then by noting the existence of the surprising 3:1 ratio. In so doing he was able to make the brilliant deduction for which genetics will be forever indebted. Though Mendel had no way of knowing it at the time, his two "gametes" are now known to be a pair of genes. A different pair of genes is involved in the determination of each trait. When more complex traits are involved, more than one pair of genes may be involved, as will be seen later on in this chapter.

This second important principle enunciated by Mendel is known as the law of independent segregation, which states that *the inheritance of one trait is independent of the inheritance of other traits,* since each gene that finds its way into the seminal cell of the progeny gets there strictly on its own, governed only by the laws of chance. This is not strictly true. Genes are strung like beads on chromosomes, each particular chromosome having the same set of genes for any given species. Man has twenty-three pairs of chromosomes. The garden pea plant has seven pairs. Mendel was incredibly lucky in that each of the gene pairs controlling the traits he studied was on separate chromosomes; otherwise he might not have been able to show that genes segregate independently. Obviously, different genes on the same chromosome are not independent of each other.

The consequences of these two laws are enormously important in understanding how genetics governs the acquisition of traits and their transmittal to the next generation. This includes not only the simple traits in garden pea plants but the sum of all traits found in all organisms that reproduce sexually. Among the several means naturally available to encourage variety among living things, sexual reproduction is perhaps the most ingenious and effective biological mechanism to promote diversity. It also insures that among the great diversity of traits passed on, there will always be some combinations that will possess a distinct survival advantage under any one of a wide range of possible environmental circumstances. Without diversity as conditions change, and they always do, the combinations of genes that were adequate for survival once would no longer be good enough, and the species would eventually disappear. This story has repeated itself many times since life emerged on this planet. *Thus it is important to realize that diversity is of the very essence of life,* and that sexual reproduction is one of the major genetic devices that make diversity possible.

Genetics would be very simple indeed if this understanding of Mendel's laws were all there is to know about it. Unfortunately it is only a small beginning in a long and fascinating discipline, which is beyond the scope of this chapter. For our purposes, however, the veil can be lifted on another aspect of genetics: the concept of multiple gene inheritance. Scientists always try to prove new concepts wrong by repeating and verifying past experiments. This is the best way to keep scientific work honest and forward moving. Work done by Josef Kölreuter in 1760, a century before Mendel, in which he crossed tall and dwarf varieties of tobacco plants (instead of pea plants) gave results that could not be explained and that later seemed to be contradicted by the experiments of Mendel. Kölreuter was a good biologist, known for his excellent experimental care, and no one was able to dispute the accuracy of his findings. What Kölreuter found was that when he crossed a tall with a dwarf parent *tobacco* plant he got progeny in the first generation that ranged between the tall and the dwarf parent tobacco plants, while the reader will recall that Mendel's first generation of *pea* plants was uniformly tall. The same thing happened in the second generation of to- bacco plants, whose heights ranged from tall to dwarf in a smooth, continuous distribution. Mendel, by contrast, found only tall and dwarf plants in the second generation in a ratio of three tall to every dwarf plant.

After the importance of Mendel's work was finally recognized, in 1900, many geneticists of the time thought that this continuous variation in the phenotypes (traits) of the progeny was due to a genetic mechanism completely different from the one discovered by Mendel, and the controversy raged for more than a decade.† But by 1910 some astute geneticists realized that perhaps the continuous variation observed in some cases could fit under Mendelian laws if one assumed that not *one* but *many* gene pairs were involved in the determination of the phenotype. And in- deed Nils Herman Nilsson-Ehle, a Swedish plant breeder, and Edward Murray East in the United States carried out classical experiments between 1910 and 1913 that proved this concept of multiple gene inheritance to be correct.

This concept was applied in 1913 by the geneticist Charles B. Davenport to the study of human skin color, in which he demon- strated that this phenotype also results from multiple gene inheritance.[2] Dr. Davenport believed that the difference be- tween white and black skin could be accounted for by not *one* but *two* pairs of genes. His most important studies were carried out on the islands of Bermuda and Jamaica, because these were ideal for his purpose; there was a great deal of intermarriage between Negro and Caucasian inhabitants of the islands, and

---

† Mendel had been aware of this problem but apparently did not fully recognize its significance.

[2] C. B. Davenport, "Heredity of Skin Color in Negro-White Crosses," *Carnegie Institute of Washington Publication* 188 (1913), pp. 1–106.

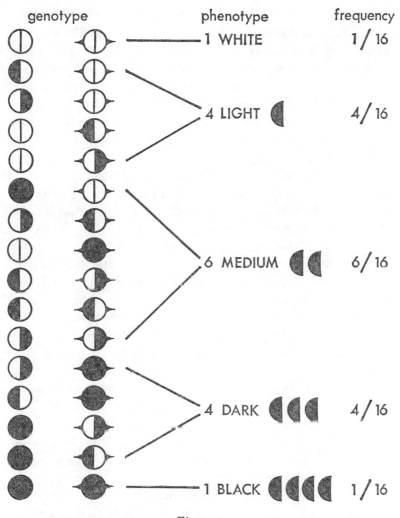

genotype	phenotype	frequency

1 WHITE   1 / 16

4 LIGHT   4 / 16

6 MEDIUM   6 / 16

4 DARK   4 / 16

1 BLACK   1 / 16

Figure 3

Illustration of the possible combinations of black and white genes
in the two-gene pairs system of Davenport for skin color

Note that there are sixteen possible combinations and that the phenotype frequency will depend on how many ways a given set of four
genes can segregate among two gene pairs. These gene pairs are shown
as circles. To emphasize that each gene pair of a set is different from
the other, little horizontal spikes appear on the circles at the right.
The 1:4:6:4:1 ratio that emerges from these calculations is exactly
what Davenport observed in a study of real populations in Jamaica
and Bermuda (see text).

very little immigration, emigration, or illegitimacy, all of which could affect the accuracy of the results.

Davenport developed an arbitrary scale of color variation from pure white (which applied to albinos, or persons totally devoid of the skin pigment melanin) at 0 per cent all the way to 100 per cent for pure black. Davenport divided his color scheme into five classes of increasing skin pigmentation: white, light, medium, dark, and black. Davenport assumed that two pairs of genes were involved. They are shown in Figure 3. According to Mendelian inheritance, these genes can exist in 16 possible combinations: 1 white, 4 light, 6 medium, 4 dark, and 1 black. And indeed Davenport was able to show an approximate ratio of 1 white for every 4 light, 6 intermediate, 4 dark, and 1 black.

Since Davenport reported his results, other scientists, notably Dr. Curt Stern, have shown that many more than two, and perhaps as many as six, pairs of genes may be involved in the determination of skin color. This complicates a careful determination of the skin-color phenotype. An additional problem is that factors such as exposure to the sun and aging cause wide variation within each phenotype and can place it in an incorrect category. But this does not change the significance of the general principle of multiple-gene inheritance developed by Nilsson-Ehle, East, and Davenport, among others. It has been abundantly demonstrated to exist in the detailed study of a wide range of phenotypes in many types of living organisms from plants to animals.

The human skin-color phenotype has been associated with many myths. The common belief that the black phenotype is dominant over the white, for instance, is without scientific foundation; white parents cannot have black children, and vice versa. Examination of Mendelian genetics in Figure 3 will make this fact abundantly clear. Recall that in each of the two pairs of genes there can be from 0 to 4 pigment genes (each black half circle) in different possible combinations, representing increasingly darker skin color. It makes no difference where the black half circles are; what counts is how many of them are present.

In other words, identical phenotypes (traits) can be produced by a large number of different genotypes.

The principle involved is the same one used by hardware stores in preparing house-paint colors. One or more preweighed packets of pigment are added to a white paint base. The more packets added, the darker the paint, according to an instruction manual followed by the paint mixer. The instruction manual and the paint packets are equivalent to the genes (genotype), while the final paint color is the trait (phenotype). Returning to Figure 3, if each parent has a genotype corresponding to only one "black gene" out of four, parents with the "light gene" each can contribute, at best, only one "black gene," so the offspring cannot carry more than two (out of four) "black genes." Therefore, the children's skin color can range from white to medium, but it cannot be darker. It must be emphasized again that many more than two pairs of genes are actually involved in the determination of the skin-color phenotype, but the principle remains the same. It is also important to point out that the genes themselves don't carry the skin pigment melanin; rather, they are the coded instructions that direct the cell to make that pigment.

The crucially important point the above discussion has intended to illustrate is this: the human skin-pigmentation phenotype is easy to recognize, observe, and measure, but its genotype is already so complex, so subject to wide variations imposed by environmental factors such as sunlight and age, that much still remains to be done before it becomes completely predictable.

If the jump is now made to another phenotype—what is called "intelligence" as determined by "intelligence tests"—the problem becomes immeasurably more difficult to study. Practically nothing is known about the genotype associated with what can be called normal human intelligence. The number of gene pairs that may be concerned with this assumed phenotype probably runs into the hundreds, and our knowledge of their influence on each other is well beyond the scope of current scientific knowledge and insight.

Even in the case of human skin pigmentation, a person with

our hypothetical, Figure 3, one-"black gene" genotype, for instance, who lives in the tropics, or a farmer working outdoors under a blazing sun, will have a darker skin than another person, a two-"black gene" genotype, who lives at a northern latitude and leads a sedentary existence. And we are dealing here with only two pairs of genes. How do we determine a possible phenotype such as intelligence, which is so elusive, so difficult to define, and whose genotype is so incredibly complex and beyond our current understanding? In other words, where exactly does the influence of genetics end and that of the environment begin? The only possible honest answer is: *we simply do not know*. But we do know that the many environmental factors interact and play a major role in modifying the phenotype, as the example of human skin-color variation under the influence of sunshine suggests.

The determination of the relative importance of heredity and environment on human behavior, in this instance of nutrition on brain development, is an extraordinarily complex endeavor, replete with pitfalls. Dr. Lancelot Hogben, best known by the public for his *Mathematics for the Million*, provides a striking imaginary example of one such pitfall with a possible consequence:[3]

It is wartime. A major city has been under siege for a long time. The blockade is complete and no food has been coming in. What is left of the food supply is deficient in several essential vitamins. As a result, the one million young children of the city are stunted, and their size and weight are significantly lower than those of the children born in that city before the war. But there is one man in the city who exercised a remarkable degree of knowledge and foresight. He is a biochemist with four children, and he managed to acquire an adequate store of pure vitamins for his family. His four children grow up normally in the besieged city.

As a result of increasing political pressure, the government appoints a high-level committee of respected individuals to de-

---

[3] L. Hogben, *Nature and Nurture*, William Withering Memorial Lectures on the Methods of Medical Genetics, 1933 (London: Allen & Unwin, 1933), p. 117.

termine whether the children are stunted because of an environmental deficiency, i.e., the diet, and if so, to sue for peace.

After careful statistical analysis, the committee reports that
only an infinitesimal proportion of the children (only 4 in 1,000,-
000) exhibit a weight variation due to a difference in the diet.
This number, they conclude, is statistically insignificant, and any
improvement in nutrition that would result from making peace
is therefore negligible. The committee report is accepted by
the government and the decision is made to continue the war.

When presented in such unequivocal terms, it is easy to see
what is wrong with the committee's reasoning. To throw a drop
of red ink into a gallon of white paint won't make much difference in the color of the paint. But adding that drop of red ink to
each and every teaspoon of white paint most assuredly will. To
divide the biochemist's vitamins among a million children will
have no effect, but to distribute a full supply to each child will.
The error consists of confusing the small effect of a measure applied only to a slight extent with the effect that a consistent measure would produce if properly applied. This type of confusion
is unfortunately only too common in the statistical analysis of
data that assess the relative importance of heredity and environment on mental capacity.

It has been estimated that the human genome, the complete
set of genes carried by each individual, consists of a total of more
than 10 million gene pairs. It is easy to study the effect of a few
genes on the resulting phenotype, whether it be a visible trait
such as skin color or a less obvious one such as the presence or
absence in the body of a substance that can be detected only by
biochemical analysis. In these cases it is often possible to make
accurate and reliable predictions of their effect on the individual
or the population. But as we deal with increasingly complex
phenotypes, the limit of our ability to draw conclusions and make
predictions is rapidly exceeded.

While some phenotypes, such as skin color, can be readily
and significantly modified by environmental factors, there are
others which are totally under genetic control. Among these is the

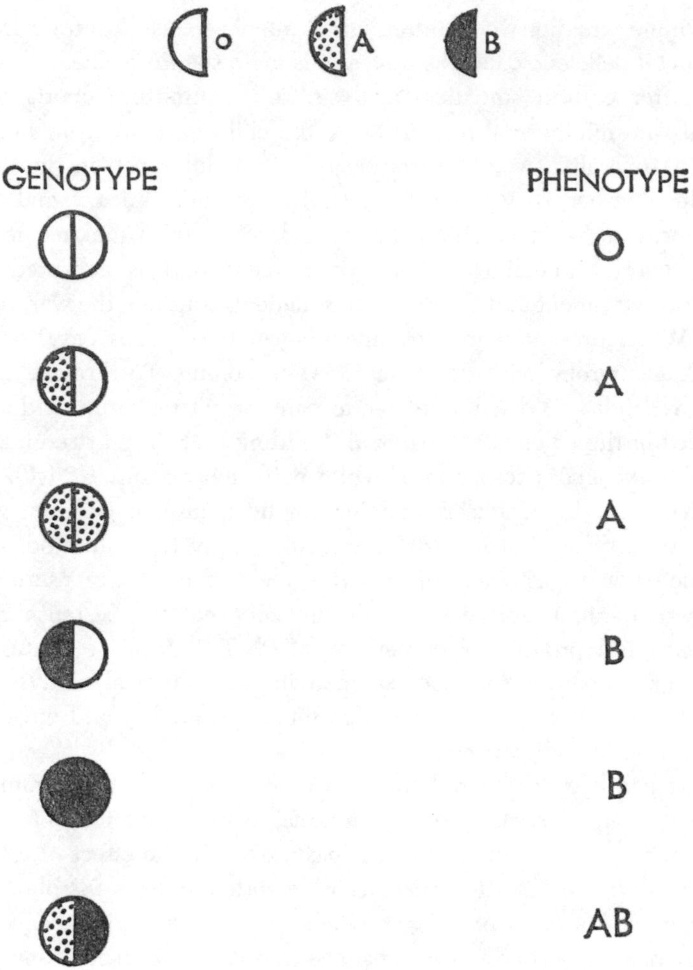

 o A B

GENOTYPE   PHENOTYPE

⟨|⟩   O

◑   A

◉   A

◐   B

●   B

◑   AB

Figure 4
Illustration of the ABO blood groups

ABO blood grouping is determined by one pair of genes, but instead
of the usual two possible genes, there are at least three: o, A, and B.
Both A and B are dominant over o in the same manner as TALL is
dominant over dwarf in Figure 1. When both dominants appear together, the stalemate is resolved by the phenotype expression of the
characteristics of both blood groups A and B.

well-known ABO blood-group phenotype, which is controlled by a single pair of genes, each gene existing in more than two configurations. These polymorphic combinations have been found to vary widely among human groups.[4] The blood groups can be identified with great accuracy, because there is a direct relationship between the genotype and the phenotype (antigens in the blood), which remains fixed for life. Figure 4 illustrates the phenotype and associated genotypes for the ABO blood groups.

One's ABO blood group is probably not influenced by environment, although certain blood-group combinations may confer survival advantage under certain circumstances and may be involved in natural selection over a period of many generations. A distribution of blood groups among world populations is shown in Table I.

An analysis of the ABO blood groups demonstrates three fundamental aspects of genetic variations involving human racial groups.

1. The extent of variation *within* any racial group generally far exceeds the average difference *between* them (see the blood-group variations among the American Indians in Table I and compare with the rest of the list).

2. The differences *between* human groups are mostly measured in *quantitative* rather than *qualitative* terms.

3. The variation between human groups is usually gradual rather than sharp at the geographical boundary between them. This arises mostly as a consequence of interaction among them.

Since these factors apply to simple phenotypes that are not influenced by environment, other phenotypes, of greater complexity, which are influenced by environment, cannot be said to apply exclusively to any one human group. Human behavior, including cognitive faculties, belongs to this category, though there are several known circumstances under which a single pair of genes may contribute to severe mental retardation. Phenylketonuria (PKU) is one such example.

---

[4] A. E. Mourant, *The Distribution of the Human Blood Groups* (Oxford: Blackwell Scientific Publications, 1954).

TABLE I

FREQUENCY OF ABO BLOOD GROUPS
IN TYPICAL POPULATIONS[5]

	O	A	B	AB
American Indians:				
Utes (Montana)	VH	VL	O	O
Toba (Argentina)	VH	VL	O	O
Sioux (South Dakota)	VH	L	VL	O
Navajo (New Mexico)	H	ML	O	O
Blackfeet (Montana)	ML	H	O	O
Shoshone (Wyoming)	MH	MH	VL	VL
Australian Aborigines (Queensland)	MH	ML	VL	O
Basques (Spain)	MH	MH	VL	O
Eskimo (Cape Farewell)	MH	MH	VL	VL
Polynesians (Hawaii)	ML	H	VL	VL
English (London)	MH	MH	L	VL
Turks (Istanbul)	ML	MH	L	L
Swedes (Stockholm)	ML	MH	L	L
Icelanders (Iceland)	MH	ML	L	L
Armenians (Turkey)	ML	MH	L	L
French (Paris)	ML	MH	L	L
Micronesians (Saipan)	MH	ML	L	L
Germans (Berlin)	ML	MH	L	L
Hungarians (Budapest)	ML	MH	L	L
Italians (Sicily)	MH	ML	L	VL
Siamese (Bangkok)	ML	L	ML	L
Lebanese (Meshghara)	ML	ML	ML	VL
Japanese (Tokyo)	ML	ML	ML	L
Russians (Moscow)	ML	ML	ML	L
Egyptians (Cairo)	ML	ML	ML	L
Pygmies (Belgian Congo)	ML	ML	ML	L
Arabs (Bedouin)	MH	ML	ML	VL
Chinese (Peking)	ML	ML	ML	L
Indians (Goa)	ML	ML	ML	L

O = none or vanishingly low (less than 0.1%)
VL = very low (less than 5%)
L = low (5 to 20%)
ML = moderately low (21 to 40%)
MH = moderately high (41 to 60%)
H = high (61 to 80%)
VH = very high (more than 80%)

---

[5] Adapted from W. C. Boyd, *Genetics and the Races of Man* (Boston: Little, Brown, 1950), p. 223.

PKU is an inherited disease belonging to a group of diseases known as inborn errors of metabolism. The disease is controlled by a single pair of genes and is expressed as the inability to metabolize (change chemically) the amino acid phenylalanine into another amino acid, tyrosine. These two amino acids are components of many proteins. This bottleneck causes a very sharp increase in the concentration of a related substance, phenylpyruvic acid, in the circulating blood, which in turn causes brain damage to the developing brain and concurrent severe mental retardation. The mechanism by which this occurs is still unknown. If PKU is detected early, however, and if a diet devoid of phenylalanine is provided during the early years of life, the extent of the brain damage can be controlled and a good mental capacity may be salvaged. In other words, the environment in this case can drastically influence the expression of the genetic factor responsible for PKU.

It is necessary at this point to say something about the meaning of that very tricky word "race." It is almost always used to define a group of human beings sociologically related. In this book, race is defined biologically. The two often coincide, but they are not synonymous. This means that members of a given human group share biological characteristics that make it possible for the group to be differentiated from another group. Thus defined, racial diversity is at the root of survival of the human species. To select one kind of genome, if that were possible, as the superior one and to act so as to discourage and eventually destroy the others would be, in effect, to put all our human eggs in one basket.

The great contemporary geneticist Dr. Theodosius Dobzhansky has pointed out that all men have been created equal, but that most certainly they are not all alike, and that the idea of equality derives from ethics, while the biological differences are observable facts. Human equality is not predicated on biological identity, nor even on identity of ability, but only on equality of opportunity. And yet, Dobzhansky continues, equality is often confused with identity, and diversity with inequality. The glaring inequalities of the rich and the poor, the powerful and the weak, the masters and the slaves, are difficult to reconcile with the idea of the universal brotherhood of man, to which many people pay lip service. An escape from this paradox is made by blaming nature or the Creator for having made some of us able and others stupid, some hard-working and others lazy.[6]

But Dobzhansky's analysis is directed to human beings as individuals, and not to racial groups. Thus the word "race" is not a clearly defined, scientific term. As popularly used, it is responsible for much confusion, misunderstanding, and human misery. Perhaps the best objective working definition of race has been made by Dobzhansky: races are populations that differ in the incidence of some genes. This definition is not based on the increasingly obsolete use of anthropological phenotypes such as skin color, skull and body shapes, and hair characteristics. Instead it implies a classification based directly on the human genomes susceptible to unequivocal biochemical or immunological identification, such as blood groups. When this is done, it becomes possible to classify human diversity into subgroups that share common sets of genes with a higher frequency than other subgroups. This is perhaps the only sensible way to look upon race.[7]

In July 1952 the United Nations Educational, Scientific and Cultural Organization (UNESCO) published a statement on race prepared by a group of internationally recognized geneticists and anthropologists. The major points made in this statement were:

1. Man belongs to a single species, *Homo sapiens*, which derived from a common stock.

2. Some of the physical differences between human groups are due to differences both of heredity and of environment.

3. National, religious, geographical, linguistic, and cultural groups do not necessarily coincide with racial groups.

---

[6] I. M. Lerner, *Heredity, Evolution and Society* (San Francisco: W. H. Freeman, 1968). This is a most interesting and lucid book by an outstanding geneticist and humanist. It is highly recommended to the reader interested in pursuing the subject in greater detail.
[7] Ibid., p. 221.

4. In general, individuals belonging to major groups are distinguishable by virtue of their physical characteristics, but individuals and small groups belonging to different races within the same major groups are usually not so easily distinguishable.

5. Innate capacity and environmental opportunity determine the results of intelligence and temperament tests.

6. Genetically determined cultural differences do not warrant popularly held notions of racial superiority or inferiority. (This point was made by UNESCO in another context in the statement.)

7. There is no evidence for the existence of so-called "pure" races. Human hybridization has been going on for a very long time.

8. Equality of opportunity and equality under the law, as ethical principles, in no way depend upon the assertion that human beings are in fact equal in endowment.

Before the advent of new biochemical and immunological determinants of racial groups, a number of sociological or cultural factors were advanced as evidence of race. They have invariably broken down under the harsh glare of scientific findings. The concept that race and language are related, for example, can be shown to be wrong. The language of Iceland is Scandinavian, but the blood groups and other genetic profile data assign its population to the Celts, whose language is strikingly different. The Jews offer perhaps the best evidence that race and religion are not related, for while they are commonly thought to be a single, clearly defined race, in actual fact the genome of the Jewish population generally coincides with that of the population surrounding it. For example, Yemenite Jews are high in blood group O and low in A and B, as are the Yemenite Arabs, while the Cochin Jews have about the same relatively high A and B groups as the Cochin Hindus.

In 1855, Joseph Arthur Comte de Gobineau, a French diplomat who served briefly under Prime Minister Alexis de Tocqueville, published the last of four volumes entitled *Essai sur l'Inégalité des Races Humaines* (Essay on the Inequality of the Human Races). The essential message of this verbose undertaking was that Aryan‡ racial purity should be preserved, that goal to be accomplished by the hereditary protection of the Nordic strains of Europe.[8]

With liberalism in eclipse in France and Germany since the revolution of 1848, and with the star of Prince Otto von Bismarck, proponent of Prussian greatness, in the ascendancy, Gobineau's concept of racial superiority found a favorable reception in aristocratic and intellectual circles of the time. Even though Gobineau himself protested against the tendentious distortion by others of what he had written, his essay proved to be powerfully influential and the enduring catalyst for the development of racial theories of the twentieth century and their tragic consequences.

Tocqueville could not accept his friend's views as scientifically sound and valid, any more than can thinking men today. In a letter to Gobineau, Tocqueville asked: "What advantage can there be in persuading base peoples living in barbarism, indolence and slavery that, such being their racial nature, they can do nothing to improve their situation or to change their habits and government? Do you not see inherent in your doctrine all the evils engendered by permanent inequality—pride, violence, scorn of fellow men, tyranny and abjection in all their forms?"[9]

Mankind has grievously suffered from the propagation of false ideologies based on ignorance or refusal to recognize the validity

---

‡ Dr. I. M. Lerner, op. cit., quotes the nineteenth-century philologist F. M. Müller, who once believed that race and language were related, but in his later years unceasingly repeated, "I have declared again and again that if I say 'Aryans' I mean neither blood nor bones nor hair nor skull. I mean those who speak an Aryan language." But the blatant misuse of the term "Aryan," a word legitimately applicable to language only, still exists today. This is part of the legacy of racism contributed to the world first by Gobineau and later by Nazi Germany.

[8] J. A. de Gobineau, The Inequality of Human Races, trans. by Adrian Collins (New York: Howard Fertig, 1967).

[9] Quoted in M. D. Biddiss, Father of Racist Ideology, The Social and Political Thought of Count Gobineau (New York: Weybright & Talley, 1970), p. 149.

of refuting evidence. Genetic principles do not support these commonly believed assertions about human populations. A given human population may possess a variety of attributes in large or small amount; but it is meaningless to state that one population is superior or inferior to another, and it is not even possible to test the validity of that assertion on genetic grounds.

Chapter IX

SCIENCE AND PUBLIC POLICY

On August 28, 1948, there appeared in the Moscow newspaper *Pravda* the text of a decree from the Presidium of the Soviet Academy of Sciences that established strict and novel guidelines for genetics research and teaching. Henceforth the "foreign" science of Mendelian genetics would be abolished, to be replaced by "Soviet" genetics, whose premise was that acquired characteristics could be inherited.

The appeal of this concept, originally propounded by the French naturalist Jean Baptiste Lamarck (1744–1829) is that it allows for the inheritance of traits developed from the experience acquired during an individual's lifetime. Thus new needs generate new habits, which in turn cause inheritable changes in the offspring. Lamarck suggested, for example, that the horns of cattle resulted from their habit of butting heads in combat, and that the webbed feet of ducks arose from their need to find food in water. While most biologists had rejected these naïve superstitions by the early 1900s, both Karl Marx and Friedrich Engels were strong supporters of Lamarckism, because it offered them the possibility of improving the human race in general, and of abolishing the profit motive in particular. So, they reasoned, would Marxism triumph in the end.

Mendelian genetics is not compatible with the inheritance of acquired characteristics. While Lamarckian genetics asserted that giraffes acquired their long necks by stretching to reach the upper leaves of a tree, and then passed on this stretched-neck trait to their progeny, Mendelian genetics explained the long necks as a result of natural selection. That is, giraffes endowed with longer necks could obtain more food than those with shorter necks. This advantage would then produce more and hardier offspring. Over the following generations, the number of long-necked giraffes would increase, and so would the length of their necks. This is today accepted as the most reasonable explanation.

Between 1936 and 1948 a violent and bitter scientific controversy raged in the Soviet Union between Mendelian and Lamarckian geneticists, culminating in 1948 in the complete victory of the Lamarckians, headed by the agronomist Trofim D. Lysenko. The 1948 decree announced the appointment of Lysenko as the virtual dictator of Soviet genetics, a power he retained until the downfall of Nikita Khrushchev, in 1964. Lysenko was instrumental in the dismissal, exile, and execution of scores of the most promising Soviet geneticists. After his dismissal, Lysenko was publicly disgraced and exposed as a charlatan whose fanaticism had led to the wholesale faking of scientific data by his disciples in order to support his false notions.

It was by then too late to undo the damage; genetics as a science had been destroyed in the Soviet Union, with consequences likely to be felt for many years to come. Among these was the repeated failure of Soviet agriculture, with consequent heavy purchases of wheat from the United States. Another was the fact that a whole generation of trained geneticists, particularly agronomists, is now missing in the Soviet Union, while some Lysenko supporters still manage to survive in high government posts.[1]

---

[1] I. M. Lerner, *Heredity, Evolution and Society* (San Francisco: W. H. Freeman, 1968), pp. 277–86. This book contains an excellent detailed analysis of the rise and fall of Lysenko.

The contribution to agricultural production of one American plant geneticist alone, Dr. Norman E. Borlaug, will dispel any lingering doubt about the dimensions of this problem. Under Dr. Borlaug's direction India and Pakistan were able to increase their wheat production by 50 per cent between 1950 and 1970. India alone recorded an increase of 11 million tons of wheat between 1965 and 1970. For these achievements Dr. Borlaug was awarded the Nobel Prize for Peace in 1970.[2]

Thus a political attempt to discredit "capitalistic" Mendelian genetics (Mendel was a priest) and arduous efforts to promote a chauvinistic science, with promises of rapid improvements in the standard of living and appeals to national pride, boomeranged with a vengeance on its instigators. They discovered, to their sorrow, that scientific knowledge is based on evidence of universal applicability whose availability transcends geographical boundaries and political or religious ideologies. In scientific matters, all attempts at suppression or control are dearly bought and must necessarily fail in the end.

Dr. Lincoln P. Bloomfield, Professor of Political Science, Massachusetts Institute of Technology, and former U. S. Foreign Service officer, recently wrote:

"The greatest single lesson for leadership, and the heart of the needed transformation in American attitudes about its world role turns on this: the air, the water, the quality of people's lives, the communications that enrich them, the wars and diseases that kill them, the consequences of affluence and scientific discovery —every single one of these will turn out on analysis to be largely indifferent to a single nation's boundaries and effectively approachable only on the basis of regional or international cooperation and eventually international regulation."[3]

The Lysenko affair is not a unique event in scientific history,

---

[2] A. Chase, *The Biological Imperatives—Health, Politics and Human Survival* (New York: Holt, Rinehart & Winston, 1971), p. 357.
[3] L. P. Bloomfield, "Foreign Policy for Disillusioned Liberals," *Foreign Policy* 9 (1972), Copyright 1972 by National Affairs, Inc. Quoted by permission.

but it is the most recent and most extensive experience whose consequences can now be readily documented. There is a danger that the inconclusive debate involving race and intelligence may also degenerate into unwise political action. Much of the tangled rhetoric associated with this controversy consists of flawed arguments by both scientists and politicians. Perhaps the best statement to date on the matter was that made by Dr. Liam Hudson, Department of Educational Sciences, Edinburgh University:

"The truth of the matter is that most of the utterances made by scientists about race and intelligence are devoid either of scientific validity or educational significance. But to acknowledge this is not to dismiss the issue out of hand. Not all who argue for the influence of human genetics are racists; not all who argue from the environmental point of view are mindless egalitarians. There exists a middle ground. . . ."[4]

It is this middle ground that this book has attempted to span by considering early-life malnutrition as one factor in the total perspective—a major environmental variable in shaping cognitive potential.

There has been an uncritical general acceptance of the postulate that blacks are inherently mentally inferior to whites, no matter what the circumstances of their infancy might have been. This view has often been expressed in nicely turned phrases that attempt to soften the impact of the message they are conveying. Considerable evidence has been accumulated that shows that blacks tend, on the average, to have lower I.Q.'s than whites. But it is not possible to draw from this kind of information the conclusion that black people are mentally inferior to whites.

I.Q. scores express individual differences on a scale of difficulty related not only to an individual's age group but also to the performance of his social group on the test. Most I.Q. tests administered to blacks have been standardized on the performance of a white population whose cultural patterns are quite different

---

[4] L. Hudson, "The Context of the Debate," in *Race and Intelligence, The Fallacies Behind the Race-I.Q. Controversy*, ed. by K. Richardson, D. Spears, and M. Richards (Baltimore: Penguin Books, 1972). Quoted by permission.

from those of any black population. Therefore, what is being measured in such tests is white ability rather than black potential. It is likely that whites taking an I.Q. test standardized on the performance of a black population would suffer the same disadvantages. But even in this comparison of black and white performance, blacks can do and have done well on white-oriented tests, as the following documented examples suggest.

In 1969 the Los Angeles Board of Education reported that the Window Hills School, a predominantly black public school, was leading the city in its mean I.Q. scores.[5]

Dr. S. P. Strickland, former Director of the National Advisory Council on the Education of Disadvantaged Children, reported on a remarkable five-year project carried out in Milwaukee, Wisconsin, by a multidisciplinary team under the direction of Dr. R. Heber, Department of Education and Child Psychology, University of Wisconsin, to learn more about the relationship between poverty and mental retardation among blacks.[6] This research team included professionals from a wide variety of specialties including psychology, psychiatry, sociology, speech therapy, and education.

The area selected for study was a black residential section of Milwaukee with the lowest median income, the greatest population density, and the most dilapidated housing in the city, the classic description of an urban slum. As expected, tests showed that it yielded a much higher percentage of mentally retarded children than did any other area of Milwaukee. The most important initial observation was that the I.Q. of the mother was the best indicator of what the I.Q. of her children would be. This had also been substantiated in the studies reported by Dr. Joaquín Cravioto and his teams.

Eighty per cent of the children with an I.Q. below 80 came from fewer than half the families, those in which the mother's

---

[5] O. Walker, "The Window Hills Story," *Integrated Education*, May–June 1970, p. 4.
[6] S. P. Strickland, "Can Slum Children Learn?" *American Education*, July 1971, pp. 3–7.

I.Q. was also below 80. Usually the father's I.Q. was also very low, but the mother's score was always the more reliable. Thus, in determining the I.Q. of the children, the disadvantageous environment appeared to be less significant than the mental capacity of the parents. The immediately obvious and superficial conclusion would have been that heredity rather than environment was the dominant cause of the observed retardation.

This explanation was challenged by an extended study of more than sixty mothers with an I.Q. of less than 70 and their newborn children, a project of the Infant Education Center, established in Milwaukee in 1966. One third of the infants remained in a control group. The other two thirds were exposed to intense rehabilitation and mental stimulation; their mothers were offered training in improved homemaking, nutrition, and baby-care techniques. Three and one half years later the difference between the control and the rehabilitated groups was dramatic: the rehabilitated group scored an average of thirty-three I.Q. points higher than the control group, with the same children exhibiting I.Q. scores as high as 135. Of equal importance, these children, rehabilitated since infancy, have since continued to learn at a rate generally better than their age mates, both white and black. Much more than heredity must have been involved in these achievements.

Other studies support the view that the cognitive performance of white and black children is comparable. Among these is the study by Dr. Robert McQueen, University of Nevada, and Dr. Browning Churn, Washoe County School District, which includes the city of Reno, Nevada.[7] This sparsely populated area contains a district in which a mixed white and black population has lived in peace and stability for nearly two generations. An amicable relationship has existed during that time among school authorities, parents, and black and white leaders.

Drs. McQueen and Churn compared the I.Q. scores, academic

---

[7] R. McQueen and B. Churn, "The Intelligence and Educational Achievement of a Matched Sample of White and Negro Students," *School and Society* 88 (1960), pp. 327–29.

achievement, and classroom behavior of seventy-one white and seventy-one black students of comparable backgrounds. Thirteen different tests were performed, including several I.Q. tests, and in only two of these were observed differences large enough to be considered barely significant. In eleven of these thirteen tests the differences in the scores obtained from white and black students were so small as to be insignificant by any statistical criterion. The conclusion reached by the investigators in this study was that they could, in effect, find no difference between the I.Q. and cognitive performance of white and black students in the district.

On September 21, 1956, *U. S. News & World Report* published a statement by Dr. Frank C. J. McGurk, Department of Psychology, Villanova University, entitled "A Scientist's Report on Race Differences." Dr. McGurk asserted that improvement in the socioeconomic status of blacks was not reflected by an increase in I.Q. scores, that these results were consistent with the conclusion that blacks did not have as good a capacity to learn as whites, and that this fact had been demonstrated again and again. The generally accepted truism of black genetic cognitive inferiority was being reinforced once more by the application of the aura of scientific authority to support a sociological and political argument.

In a sharply worded challenge to Dr. McGurk's statement, Drs. William M. McCord, Stanford University, and Nicholas J. Demerath III, Harvard University, published a point-by-point rebuttal, supported by documented scientific evidence, to discredit the vague generalities of Dr. McGurk's statement in *U. S. News & World Report*.[8] The substance of this rebuttal has already been discussed in various sections of this book, but one particularly significant study reported by Drs. McCord and Demerath deserves detailed examination now. Between 1938 and 1945, 612 predelinquent and normal white and black boys were examined

---

[8] W. M. McCord and N. J. Demerath III, "Negro Versus White Intelligence: A Continuing Controversy," *Harvard Educational Review* 28 (1958), pp. 120–35.

as part of the "Cambridge-Somerville Youth Study." Under carefully controlled and matched conditions, both the Kuhlman-Anderson (group I.Q.) and Stanford-Binet (individual I.Q.) tests were given, and socioeconomic as well as genetic factors were evaluated statistically. In no case could the investigators find any significant difference in cognitive ability between white and black boys.

Dr. Eli Ginzberg, Director, Conservation of Human Resources Project, Columbia University, reported that during World War II 15,850,000 white and 2,150,000 black men were examined for military service. The low average mental aptitude of black soldiers obscured the fact that a considerable number of them scored well above the average for white soldiers. About fifty thousand blacks were classified in the two highest categories, which made them eligible for officer-training schools.[9]

In 1970 the Virginia State Board of Education reported that one of its black schools had the highest average I.Q. of any school in that state.[10]

Dr. Jane R. Mercer, Department of Sociology, University of California at Riverside, spent eight years studying the social processes by which persons become labeled as mental retardates by schools and other community organizations in Riverside, a city with a population of 130,000. She found that four times more Mexican Americans and three times more blacks were being so labeled than whites, with I.Q. tests being relied on heavily in making such diagnoses. These proportions were the same in other school districts in the state of California. Dr. Mercer noted that Mexican Americans and blacks labeled as mental retardates were less subnormal than the retarded whites and had a higher average I.Q. and fewer physical disabilities. Members of minorities were more likely to be diagnosed as retarded than whites, and for less reason. But when environmental differences were

---

[9] E. Ginzberg, *The Negro Potential* (New York: Columbia University Press, 1956), pp. 66–67.
[10] Virginia State Board of Education, *Test Score Reports, City and County Districts*, 1971.

evaluated among 6,907 Mexican Americans, blacks, and whites, Dr. Mercer found that the proportion of mental retardates, as measured by clinical standards, was comparable.[11]

In 1969 the National Merit Scholarship Corporation reported that the more than thirty per year black recipients of its coveted awards attained an average score on its examinations exceeding the 98th percentile in comparison with national norms for whites.[12]

The many children fathered by U.S. soldiers stationed abroad have proved fruitful material for investigation of racial I.Q. differences. In Germany, Dr. Von Klaus Eyferth found no difference in the I.Q. of children of black soldiers and those of their all-German counterparts.[13]

Drs. Viola Theman and Paul Witty, School of Education, Northwestern University, reported case studies of two black children in the genius class, one of whom reached 200, one of the highest scores ever recorded on an I.Q. test.[14]

In a classic study, Dr. Otto Klineberg, Columbia University, analyzed black migration from South to North since the Civil War, and more particularly since World War I.[15] The famous Alpha test given to World War I U. S. Army recruits provided the first significant opportunity to assess the I.Q.'s of blacks and whites from different regions of the United States. As Dr. Audrey M. Shuey reported later, whites scored consistently better than blacks on these white-standardized tests.[16] But another fact that

[11] J. R. Mercer and W. C. Brown, "Racial Differences in I.Q.: Fact or Artifact," in *The Fallacy of I.Q.*, ed. by C. Senna (New York: Third Press, 1973), p. 56.
[12] National Merit Scholarship Corporation Research Reports, *Outstanding Negro High School Graduates,* The Corporation, 1969.
[13] V. K. Eyferth, "Eine Untersuchung der Neger-Mischlingskinder in Westdeutchland," *Vita Humana* 2 (1959), pp. 102–14.
[14] V. Theman and P. Witty, "Case Studies and Genetic Records of Gifted Negroes," *Journal of Psychology* 15 (1943), pp. 165–81.
[15] O. Klineberg, *Negro Intelligence and Selective Migration* (New York: Columbia University Press, 1935), 64 pp.
[16] A. M. Shuey, *The Testing of Negro Intelligence,* 2nd ed. (New York: Social Science Press, 1965), p. 1.

emerged from this period was that northern blacks performed in these tests in a way clearly superior to that of southern blacks. There are two possible explanations for this geographic difference. One is that environmental opportunities available to blacks in the North were clearly superior to those in the South; these included better schools, better nutrition, and a more stimulating urban, rather than a generally more backward rural, environment. Since I.Q. tests reflect cultural and educational patterns, the higher score obtained by northern blacks could be accounted for in large part by this observation.

However, it has also been argued that it was the more intelligent blacks who migrated North to seek better opportunities than were available to them in the South, leaving their less well-endowed brethren behind, thus explaining the higher I.Q. scores of northern as compared with southern blacks. If the first of these two explanations is correct, it would suggest that environment rather than heredity is at the root of the distinct difference in the I.Q. scores of northern and southern blacks. If the northern environment is more favorable than the southern one for blacks, the evidence could demonstrate that the native ability was there from the beginning but that the opportunity to express it had to await a more suitable environment. But if the more intelligent of the southern blacks moved North, this selective migration would suggest that heredity rather than environment was the dominant factor in the relatively poorer I.Q. performance of black recruits. Their performance in the Army Alpha test of World War I would, therefore, reflect no environmental effects on mental ability but only a redistribution of northern and southern blacks.

This is the question Dr. Klineberg sought to resolve in his exhaustive analysis of the problem. Slavery, which was responsible for bringing blacks to this continent, has not been associated with primitive societies but rather with the development of agriculture and industry. In primitive societies, which usually depended on hunting, the vanquished enemy was slain rather than enslaved.

It was only when the heavy toil of land cultivation became important that the militarily weaker were exploited for their labor as slaves by the victors. Because of the immense economic advantage of this source of labor, every effort was made to protect the *status quo* so that those in bondage would never be in a position either to clearly assess or to challenge their status. Thus slavery is a universal and perhaps an inevitable stage in the development of agriculture. During the period of the industrial revolution of the nineteenth century another form of slavery arose, marked by appalling conditions of working men, women, and children. Slavery existed legally until 1942 in Ethiopia and 1962 in Saudi Arabia.[17]

In the United States many slaves escaped to the North before the Civil War, mostly through the famous Underground Railroad, and settled in northern states. In 1879 a significant migration, primarily to Kansas, of freed slaves from the South took place, followed in 1888 and subsequent years by large movements to Texas and adjoining states. By 1910 there were more than 1 million blacks in the northern states.[18] But the massive migration of blacks to the North occurred between 1915 and 1918, in response to increased demands for unskilled industrial and mining labor mainly because of World War I, together with sharply decreased immigration of European laborers.

This black migration became so extensive that it was noticed in the press in a manner that reflected the bias of the editors. Southern black papers complained that they were losing their best men, while southern white papers tried to reassure their readers that only the most undesirable blacks were migrating North. Both the black and the white northern press viewed this massive influx with alarm and were frequently hostile to the newcomers, representing them as an inferior group of human beings. These views, however, were not universal, and a considerable

---

[17] "Slavery," Encyclopaedia Britannica, Vol. 20, (Chicago: Encyclopaedia Britannica Press, 1965), pp. 786–87.
[18] O. Klineberg, *Negro Intelligence and Selective Migration* (New York: Columbia University Press, 1935), p. 6.

degree of tolerance was exhibited at the time, which probably further encouraged this northern migration. The Boston *Transcript* of March 9, 1917, for example, carried the following statement: "It takes some enterprise and resolution for a Negro to emigrate from the south to the north; those who come have probably for the most part made up their minds to struggle and adapt themselves."[19]

In New York City Dr. Klineberg made an exhaustive study of school records and I.Q.-test performance of various groups of migrants who had resided in the North for up to twelve years. He then compared these scores with those of blacks who remained in southern states. These test scores were used to determine whether the improved northern environment had any effect in raising the I.Q. scores of southern-born children. If environment had an effect, the improved I.Q. scores should reflect the length of residence in the northern environment; i.e., the longer the migrant had been in New York City, the higher his I.Q. should be. If, on the other hand, the superiority of these New York City migrants was due to selective migration, length of residence should have very little or no effect. Group I.Q. tests were also given to 1,697 twelve-year-old children in the Harlem schools during 1931–32. The results showed a clear-cut improvement in I.Q. scores with increased length of residence, supporting the environmental hypothesis. Table I summarizes one of these studies.

TABLE I[20]

Years of Residence in North	Average I.Q. City-born Children	Country-born Children
1–2	76	50
3–4	81	67
5–6	94	84
7–8	99	104
9–11	103	101

[19] Ibid., p. 8.
[20] Ibid., p. 32.

The combined results of the three studies with a total of 1,697 twelve-year-old children are summarized in Table II.

TABLE II[21]

Years of Residence in North	Average Score
1–2	72
3–4	76
5–6	84
7–8	90
9 and over	94
12 (northern born)	92

Similar results were obtained from individually given Stanford-Binet tests. A consistent relationship between length of northern residence and I.Q was found.

The segregated schools in the South were grossly inadequate to the task of educating black children. The resources available to black schools compared to white schools were pitiful. Klineberg quotes a documented account of the wide disparity in per-capita expenditure for white and black children in the southern states in the late 1920s as follows:[22]

PER-CAPITA EXPENDITURE FOR EDUCATION
IN SOUTHERN STATES (LATE 1920S)

	White School	Black School
South Carolina	$45.45	$ 4.48
Alabama	37.63	5.45
Georgia	35.24	7.44
Louisiana	42.17	9.34
Virginia	54.21	14.86
U.S.A. as a whole	$87.22	

The school handicap reflected the general status of blacks in the South. There are no records from that period describing nutritional status, but voluminous anecdotal information exists

---

[21] O. Klineberg, *Negro Intelligence and Selective Migration* (New York: Columbia University Press, 1935), p. 40.
[22] Ibid., p. 57.

that suggests malnutrition was rampant. Breast feeding, however, probably mitigated the effects of early-life malnutrition.

By contrast, the higher wages and better schools of the richer, northern states provided better opportunities for the migrant blacks than had existed in the poorer, southern states. The low I.Q. scores obtained by southern blacks and recent migrants *also* were the result of economic conditions, which forced these children to begin their schooling considerably later than white children. The poorer the environment, the longer the delay before schooling was begun.[23]

Finally Klineberg attacked the vicious and long-standing argument that the achievement level of blacks was related to the amount of white intermixture in their ancestry, a greater opportunity for which might have existed in the North than in the South. Klineberg quoted from a study of 306 twelve-year-old boys in which three negroid characteristics were used as a measure of intermixture with whites: skin color, lip thickness, and nose width, as determined by standardized measurement methods. A comparison of these three characteristics was made between two groups of children: southern-born children one to eleven years of age in northern residence, and twelve-year-olds born in the North. A summary of these data is given below:[24]

Average black skin color	(%)	29.4	± 2.85*
Average lip thickness	(mm)	21.0	± 1.95
Average nose width	(mm)	36.15	± 1.67

The table shows that there is no apparent relationship between the extent of these negroid characteristics and the length of northern residence, and therefore no evidence of change in the

---

[23] Ibid.
[24] Ibid., p. 61.
* Calculated by the author from data in Klineberg, op. cit., p. 61, Table 34. The number following the ± sign above is called the standard deviation, a measure of how much scatter there is on either side of the average value. The larger the standard deviation the greater the deviation from the average value. In this instance the standard deviation is very small.

amount of black-white intermixture by these criteria. Therefore the degree of I.Q. improvement observed in northern black migrants as the length of northern residence was increased could not be ascribed to a higher proportion of genetic characteristics associated with northern whites.

The evidence collected by Klineberg suggests that environmental improvements, rather than selective migration, played the most significant role in improving the I.Q. scores of blacks migrating from South to North. Those significant improvements further suggested that blacks could not be said to be genetically handicapped in comparison with whites.

Klineberg was a self-acknowledged environmentalist, and his work has been criticized on the grounds that he did not have adequate controls and did not limit himself to one given population of blacks migrating from South to North. Rather, he analyzed different groups of migrants, whose relationship to each other and to southern blacks has been questioned. When the evidence is considered as a whole, however, it is difficult to confer upon the white racial groups genetically acquired advantages in cognition over blacks. The observation of significant differences in average intelligence is much more likely to be the result of environmental rather than genetic inequalities.

None of what has been asserted here should be interpreted to mean that the genetic contribution to intelligence is negligible. Heredity plays a major role in the determination of cognitive potential. Modern man, of whatever skin color, probably emerged from a single ancestor and eventually spread over all the land masses of the planet. Only a few descendant lines survived the severe hurdles of evolution. These robust descendants must have possessed a high level of mental ability to seek food and shelter, to survive, and to prosper. Thus, whether modern man is white-, brown-, yellow-, or black-skinned, the chances are overwhelming that he generally has high cognitive potential. Any differences between racial groups in this respect are more likely to have arisen from genetic isolation through the ages than from any factor to which a value judgment of superiority or inferiority could be ascribed. Food has always played a critical role in human survival, and nutrition has long been used as a political weapon for human control. Manipulation of the environment through food denial was intuitively recognized by politicians as a powerful weapon long before the consequences of early-life malnutrition were understood. And there is good evidence for differential response to environmental variables among racial groups.

The effect of environmental variables on I.Q. scores has been brilliantly analyzed by Dr. Sandra Scarr-Salapatek, Institute of Child Development, University of Minnesota. She has shown that the relative contribution of heredity and environment to I.Q. scores is not a fixed value but may vary considerably from one human population group to another. Differences in social class, life style, customs of raising children, and nutritional practices all affect the extent to which heredity and environment contribute to I.Q.[25]

Even Dr. Arthur R. Jensen admits that all major studies in this field have been based on the observation of European and North American populations, and that knowledge of intelligence in different racial and cultural groups within these populations (e.g., black populations in the United States) is nonexistent.[26]

Dr. William B. Shockley's proposal to resolve that issue through a major study to be sponsored by the National Academy of Sciences is as unwise as it is unrealistic. To study this problem would require that thousands of blacks be compelled to adopt white children at birth, and vice versa, with continued intrusions for years on the privacy of the mixed families in order to record scientific data.

And what would be the practical effect of this knowledge? If the answer were that there are no racial group differences but only individual differences, the argument would be laid to rest,

[25] S. Scarr-Salapatek, "Race, Social Class and I.Q.," *Science* 174 (1971), pp. 1285–95.
[26] A. R. Jensen, "How Much Can We Boost I.Q. and Scholastic Achievement?" *Harvard Educational Review* 39 (1969), p. 64.

not for all time but for a few years at least. But if the data should disclose hereditary differences in the cognitive endowment of different racial groups, this should make no political difference in a nation conceived in freedom, equality, and justice. In neither case would anything of lasting value be gained, since the purpose of the study would be social and political rather than scientific.

Dr. Jensen rhetorically asks, "Why has there been such uniform failure of compensatory programs wherever they have been tried? What has gone wrong? In other fields, when bridges do not stand, when aircraft do not fly, when machines do not work, when treatments do not cure . . . one begins to question the basic assumptions, principles, theories and hypotheses that guide one's efforts."[27]

Yet these basic assumptions, principles, theories, and hypotheses must be sound, because bridges do stand, aircraft do fly, machines do work, and treatments do cure. The argument that the evidence for the effect of early-life malnutrition on cognitive potential is still not convincing enough to deserve attention and prompt action is rebutted by the example of the Hungarian physician Ignaz P. Semmelweis (1818–65).

Puerperal infection had been the scourge of the maternity hospitals of Europe since the Middle Ages. Even though most women delivered their babies at home, some had to be hospitalized for obstetrical complications or other reasons. Among those hospitalized, the mortality rate due to puerperal infection was one in four. The cause of this killing disease was unknown, and so was the germ theory of disease. Dr. Semmelweis became interested in the problem while still a medical student in Vienna, and investigated it in the face of vigorous opposition by the chief of maternity at the hospital. Painstakingly collecting clinical information, he concluded that the infection was being spread by the medical students themselves, going from the pathology dis-

[27] A. R. Jensen, "How Much Can We Boost I.Q. and Scholastic Achievement?" *Harvard Educational Review* 39 (1969), p. 3.

secting room, where they handled the bodies of dead mothers, directly to the labor room to examine healthy mothers. Dr. Semmelweis persuaded his colleagues and medical students to wash their hands thoroughly before examining women in labor. As a result, the mortality rate of mothers in his hospital division dropped dramatically. But Dr. Semmelweis was denied promotion to Assistant Professor and was driven from Vienna by his jealous and ignorant chief, who refused to accept the validity of the evidence.

Even though Dr. Semmelweis was later appointed to the maternity department of the hospital at Pest, Hungary, and was able to quickly lower the puerperal-infection mortality rate to less than 1 per cent, his doctrine was not accepted by the medical profession during his lifetime, because evidence supporting it was indirect and incomplete. In the meantime the lives of countless young mothers were lost in the maternity wards of European hospitals.

Today the evidence supporting a relationship between malnutrition and brain development is far better than that which Dr. Semmelweis had to back up his pioneering efforts. But it, too, is indirect and incomplete. And early-life malnutrition continues to devastate the mental potential of the afflicted poor.

Yet the *scientific* solution to this problem is as simple as washing hands to avoid transmitting infectious diseases. It lies in insuring an adequate diet for every pregnant woman, infant, and young child. But the practical application of this simple solution is greatly complicated by the ignorance of politicians, who hold the power to act.

Scientists tend to be introverted and by definition not given to advocacy. Therein lies one of the great dilemmas of our times. Even in the face of overwhelming factual support for a given position, scientists are reluctant to speak with a single voice, lest the position they take eventually be proved wrong. Scientific discoveries cannot be made without this attitude of general skepticism and humility before the evidence. Still, the scientist must speak out in clear and unequivocal language in order to inform and educate the citizens and their political representatives at all levels of government. No one else can perform this vital task for him. The position of the scientist in our society has changed dramatically in recent years; the once-obscure, solitary investigator has become a public figure, supported at public expense, who commands tools able to change the course of human existence.

Early-life malnutrition is a probable cause of brain deficiencies. The problem is now a social one for which a scientific solution exists. Implementation of that solution lies where social priorities are established: in the political sphere.

Scientific knowledge is not of itself good or evil. It is in the wisdom of its application that the fate of mankind will continue to be determined.

INDEX